Math and Dosage Calculations for Health Occupations

Math and Dosage Calculations for Health Occupations

Renee A. Dawe
Director of Training
Health Care Properties
Red Bank, New Jersey

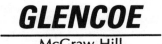

GLENCOE
McGraw-Hill

New York, New York   Columbus, Ohio   Mission Hills, California   Peoria, Illinois

This textbook has been prepared with the assistance of Voltex Corp.

Printed in the United States of America.

Send all inquires to:
Glencoe/McGraw-Hill
936 Eastwind Drive
Westerville, OH 43081

ISBN 0-02-800677-1

2 3 4 5 6 7 8 9 10   CUS   99 98 97 96 95

TABLE OF CONTENTS

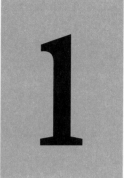

Common Fractions

PART 1: INTRODUCTION TO COMMON FRACTIONS

OBJECTIVES

1. *Identify a common fraction.*
2. *Express the meaning of a common fraction in three ways.*

A number that expresses the relationship of one or more equal parts to the total number of equal parts in one unit (or one group) is called a fraction. Fractions are important; sometimes buying a whole pizza is out of the question, but paying for half of a pizza is possible. Fractions are a way of looking at parts of a whole, whether it is a pizza or part of a vial of medicine. The **common fraction** consists of two numerals, one above the other, separated by a fraction bar.

The Meaning of a Common Fraction

A COMMON FRACTION is:

PART OF A WHOLE NUMBER

The fraction $\frac{2}{3}$ (two-thirds) means that 2 out of 3 equal parts in one whole are being considered.

ONE NUMBER DIVIDED BY ANOTHER

The fraction $\frac{2}{3}$ (two-thirds), read from top to bottom, means 2 divided by 3, $2 \div 3$, or $3\overline{)2}$.

A PRODUCT OF MULTIPLICATION

The fraction $\frac{2}{3}$ (two-thirds) means that there are 2 of the thirds, or $(2 \times \frac{1}{3})$.

When a *single thing* (unit) is divided into equal parts, a fraction shows the relationship between part of the whole and the whole.

$\frac{3}{4}$ of the square is shaded.
$\frac{1}{4}$ of the square is not shaded.
$\frac{4}{4}$ is one whole square.

When a *group of things* is divided into equal parts, a fraction shows the relationship between some of the equal parts and all of the equal parts in one whole group.

$\frac{3}{5}$ of the group is shaded.

$\frac{2}{5}$ of the group is not shaded.

$\frac{5}{5}$ is one whole group.

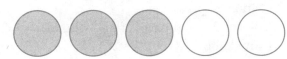

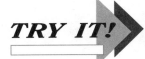 **PRACTICE**

Express each of the following fractions in three different ways.

1. $\frac{3}{4}$

   _____

   _____

   _____

2. $\frac{1}{2}$

   _____

   _____

   _____

3. $\frac{3}{8}$

   _____

   _____

   _____

4. Write a fraction that tells:
   what part of the circle is shaded. _____ ($\frac{2}{3}$)
   what part of the circle is unshaded. _____ ($\frac{1}{3}$)
   $\frac{3}{3}$ is a whole circle.

5. Write a fraction that tells:

what part of the group is shaded. _____ $(\frac{5}{7})$

what part of the group is unshaded. _____ $(\frac{2}{7})$

$\frac{7}{7}$ is one whole group.

ADDITIONAL PRACTICE

Write fractions to express the shaded portion and unshaded portion of each unit or group.

6. Shaded portion of the group _____

Unshaded portion of the group _____

$\frac{4}{4}$ is 1 whole group.

7. Shaded portion of the rectangle _____

Unshaded portion of the rectangle _____

$\frac{8}{8}$ is 1 whole rectangle.

8. Shaded portion of the circle _____

Unshaded portion of the circle _____

$\frac{8}{8}$ is 1 whole circle.

9. Shaded portion of the group _____

Unshaded portion of the group _____

$\frac{9}{9}$ is 1 whole group.

10. Shaded portion of the square _____

Unshaded portion of the square _____

$\frac{4}{4}$ is 1 whole square.

PART 2: DENOMINATOR, NUMERATOR, AND FRACTION BAR

OBJECTIVES

1. *Identify the two terms of a fraction.*
2. *State two pieces of information obtained from the denominator.*
3. *State one piece of information obtained from the numerator.*

A common fraction has a **denominator,** a **numerator** and a **fraction bar.** The denominator and the numerator are called **the terms of the fraction.** The fraction bar represents the operation of division.

Denominator

A **d**enominator (**d**own below the fraction bar) gives two very important pieces of information.

The DENOMINATOR tells:

the TOTAL number of EQUAL parts in ONE whole the SIZE of each equal part in one whole

In the fraction $\frac{2}{3}$, the denominator of 3 means 3 equal parts in one whole the size of each part is one third ($\frac{1}{3}$)

In the fraction $\frac{1}{2}$, the denominator of 2 means 2 equal parts in one whole the size of each part is one half ($\frac{1}{2}$)

3 If the denominator is 3, it means that one whole has 3 equal parts and each part has the size of one-third ($\frac{1}{3}$). Then $\frac{2}{3}$ is read "two-thirds."

2 If the denominator is 2, it means that one whole has 2 equal parts and each part has the size of one-half ($\frac{1}{2}$). Then $\frac{2}{2}$ is read "two-halves."

1 If the denominator is 1, it means that one whole has 1 equal part and that part has the size of one whole. Then $\frac{2}{1}$ is read "two wholes."

0 **The denominator of a fraction can never be zero.** It is impossible for zero parts to make one whole and it is impossible to divide by zero.

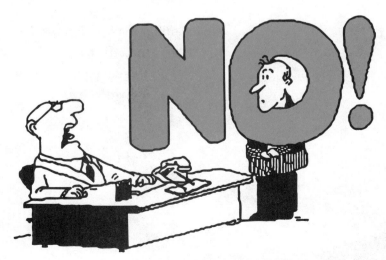

The denominator of a fraction can never be zero.

- A larger denominator means that one whole has been divided into more parts, so the pieces are a smaller size.
- A smaller denominator means that one whole has been divided into fewer parts, so the pieces are a larger size.
- **The denominator can have any value except for zero.** Zero parts could never make up one whole. It is impossible to divide by zero.

Numerator

A numerator (**up** above the fraction bar) gives one important piece of information.

The NUMERATOR tells the NUMBER of EQUAL parts being used, talked about, or considered

In the fraction $\frac{2}{3}$, the numerator of 2 means that 2 equal parts are being talked about or used (out of a total of 3 equal parts in one whole).

$\frac{2}{3}$ of the rectangle is shaded.
$\frac{1}{3}$ of the rectangle is not shaded.
$\frac{3}{3}$ is one whole rectangle.

Fraction Bar

In mathematics, the symbol ($\div$) means "divided by." Think of the fraction bar as the same symbol, except with the dots replaced by numerals. The fraction is thus an expression of division.

Read a fraction from top to bottom when reading it as an expression of division.

$$\frac{7}{8} = 7 \text{ divided by } 8 \quad = 7 \div 8 \quad = 8\overline{)7}$$

$$\frac{4}{4} = 4 \text{ divided by } 4 \quad = 4 \div 4 \quad = 4\overline{)4}$$

$$\frac{10}{5} = 10 \text{ divided by } 5 = 10 \div 5 = 5\overline{)10}$$

The meaning of a fraction can be expressed in many different ways.

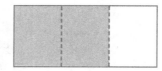

three-fifths
3 equal parts out of a total of 5 equal parts in one whole
3 divided by 5
$3 \div 5$
$5\overline{)3}$
3 of the fifths ($3 \times \frac{1}{5}$)

TRY IT!

PRACTICE

Examine the following fractions. Write the answers on the lines provided.

1. In the fraction $\frac{5}{6}$, the denominator is _____. This denominator means that there are _____ equal parts in one whole. The size of each part is a _____.

2. In the fraction $\frac{5}{6}$, the numerator is _____. This number means that _____ equal parts are being talked about or considered.

3. The fraction $\frac{2}{2}$ is read "_____ - _____." It means _____ ÷ _____.

4. The fraction $\frac{6}{1}$ is read "_____-_____" and means _____ ÷ _____.

ANSWERS

1. The denominator—down below the fraction bar—is 6. This means there are 6 equal parts in one whole. The size of each part is a sixth or $\frac{1}{6}$.
2. The numerator is 5. 5 equal parts are being talked about or considered.
3. $\frac{2}{2}$ = two halves = 2 ÷ 2 = 1
4. $\frac{6}{1}$ = six wholes = 6 ÷ 1 = 6

ADDITIONAL PRACTICE

Fill in the blanks about each fraction.

Look at the fraction $\frac{3}{4}$.

5. What is the total number of equal parts in 1 whole? _____
6. What is the size of each part? _____
7. How many parts are being talked about or used? _____
8. The numerator is _____.
9. The denominator is _____.

Look at the fraction $\frac{4}{4}$.

10. What is the total number of equal parts in 1 whole? _____
11. What is the size of each part? _____
12. How many parts are being talked about or used? _____
13. The numerator is _____.
14. The denominator is _____.

Look at the fraction $\frac{7}{4}$.

15. What is the total number of equal parts in 1 whole? _____
16. What is the size of each part? _____
17. How many parts are being talked about or used? _____
18. The numerator is _____.
19. The denominator is _____.

OBJECTIVES

1. *Identify proper and improper fractions.*
2. *State the value of any common fraction as equal to one, less than one, or greater than one.*

There are two kinds of common fractions: **proper fractions** and **improper fractions**. Proper fractions have a value that is less than one, while improper fractions have a value that is equal to one or greater than one.

Proper Fractions

A proper fraction has a numerator that is smaller than the denominator. The value of a proper fraction is less than one.

The fraction $\frac{3}{4}$ means that 3 equal parts out of four equal parts in one whole are being used. $\frac{3}{4}$ is less than one whole circle.

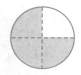

The fraction $\frac{4}{5}$ means that 4 equal parts out of 5 equal parts in one whole group are being used. $\frac{4}{5}$ is less than one whole group.

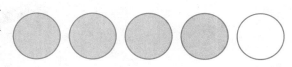

So $\frac{3}{4}$ and $\frac{4}{5}$ are examples of proper fractions. The numerator is smaller than the denominator in each case, and each fraction is less than one.

Improper Fractions

An improper fraction has a numerator that is equal to or greater than the denominator. The value of an improper fraction is equal to one or greater than one. $\frac{4}{4}$, $\frac{5}{1}$, and $\frac{7}{4}$ are examples of improper fractions.

A. **When the numerator and denominator are equal, the fraction is equal to one.**

$\frac{4}{4}$ = 4 fourths

Means one whole consists of 4 equal parts. Each part is a fourth.

We are considering 4 of those fourths.

$\frac{4}{4}$ = 4 ÷ 4 = 1 whole square.

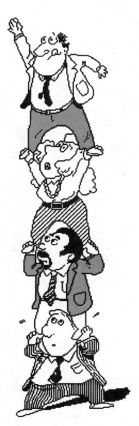

4/4 means that this one whole stack of persons consists of 4 equal parts. Each would-be acrobat is a fourth of the stack. 4/4 is 4 divided by 4 and equals 1 (stack). Harry on the bottom is holding 3 out of the 4 persons in the stack or 3/4 of the stack. Harry's not too bright.

Here are more examples of fractions that are equal to one.

$\frac{5}{5}$ = 5 divided by 5   = 5 ÷ 5   = 1 $\frac{5}{5}$ = 1

$\frac{9}{9}$ = 9 divided by 9   = 9 ÷ 9   = 1 $\frac{9}{9}$ = 1

$\frac{20}{20}$ = 20 divided by 20 = 20 ÷ 20 = 1 $\frac{20}{20}$ = 1

B. When the denominator is 1, the fraction is equal to the whole number in the numerator.

$\frac{5}{1}$ = 5 wholes   Means one whole consists of 1 equal part. Each part is a whole.

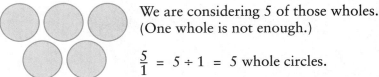

We are considering 5 of those wholes. (One whole is not enough.)

$\frac{5}{1}$ = 5 ÷ 1 = 5 whole circles.

C. When the numerator is greater than the denominator, the fraction equals more than one.

$\frac{7}{4}$ = 7 fourths

Means one whole consists of 4 equal parts. Each part is a fourth.

We are considering 7 of those fourths. (There aren't enough fourths in one whole. More fourths are needed from another square.)
7 fourths is one whole and $\frac{3}{4}$ of another whole.

$$\frac{7}{4} = 7 \div 4 = 1\frac{3}{4}$$

$1\frac{3}{4}$ is called a mixed number because it is a "mixture" of a whole number and a fraction.

Here are more examples of fractions that are equal to more than one.

$\frac{5}{3}$ = 5 thirds = 5 divided by 3 = 5 ÷ 3 = $1\frac{2}{3}$

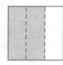

$\frac{8}{4}$ = 8 fourths = 8 divided by 4 = 8 ÷ 4 = 2

$\frac{21}{5}$ = 21 fifths = 21 divided by 5 = 21 ÷ 5 = $4\frac{1}{5}$

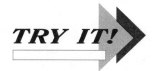

PRACTICE

Fill in the chart for each fraction.

FRACTION	WORDS	TYPE (proper or improper)	EXPRESSION OF DIVISION
EXAMPLE $\frac{10}{10}$	ten-tenths	improper	$10 \div 10$
1. $\frac{8}{7}$			
2. $\frac{3}{7}$			
3. $\frac{7}{7}$			

ANSWERS

1. Eight-sevenths is an improper fraction, $8 \div 7$
2. Three-sevenths is a proper fraction, $3 \div 7$
3. Seven-sevenths is an improper fraction, $7 \div 7$

ADDITIONAL PRACTICE

Fill in the chart for each fraction.

FRACTION	WORDS	TYPE (proper or improper)	EXPRESSION OF DIVISION
EXAMPLE $\frac{4}{1}$	4 wholes	improper	$4 \div 1$
4. $\frac{2}{2}$			
5. $\frac{7}{2}$			
6. $\frac{1}{2}$			
7. $\frac{10}{1}$			
8. $\frac{1}{1}$			
9. $\frac{9}{4}$			
10. $\frac{3}{4}$			
11. $\frac{5}{5}$			
12. $\frac{9}{7}$			
13. $\frac{7}{8}$			

	FRACTION	WORDS	TYPE (proper or improper)	EXPRESSION OF DIVISION
14.	$\frac{5}{3}$			
15.	$\frac{1}{10}$			
16.	$\frac{4}{2}$			
17.	$\frac{3}{3}$			
18.	$\frac{9}{10}$			

◆◆◆◆◆◆ **FUN FACTS** ◆◆◆◆◆◆

Of the 206 bones in the human body, one fourth or twenty-five percent of them are in the feet.

PART 4: EQUIVALENT FRACTIONS

OBJECTIVES

1. *Build a set of equivalent fractions.*
2. *Reduce a common fraction to lowest terms.*

Fractions which have the same value, but look different, are called **equivalent (equal) fractions.** The written form of the fractions change, but the value of the fractions remain the same.

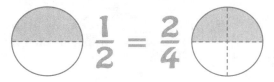

Building a Set of Equivalent Fractions

Building a set of equivalent fractions is like a game. The game must be played "fairly." The numerator and denominator must be treated in exactly the same way.

If the numerator and denominator are each *multiplied* by the same number, an equivalent fraction is created. (Any number, that is, except zero.)

$$\frac{1 \times 2 = 2}{2 \times 2 = 4}$$

A set of five fractions equal to $\frac{1}{3}$ can be made by multiplying the numerator and denominator each by the same number.

$$\left.\begin{array}{l} \dfrac{1 \times 2 = 2}{3 \times 2 = 6} \\[1.2em] \dfrac{1 \times 3 = 3}{3 \times 3 = 9} \\[1.2em] \dfrac{1 \times 4 = 4}{3 \times 4 = 12} \\[1.2em] \dfrac{1 \times 5 = 5}{3 \times 5 = 15} \end{array}\right\} \text{ all equal } \frac{1}{3} \; \left(\frac{1}{3}, \frac{2}{6}, \frac{3}{9}, \frac{4}{12}, \frac{5}{15}\right)$$

It is possible, of course, to make more fractions equal to $\frac{1}{3}$. Multiply the numerator and denominator each by 6, multiply the numerator and denominator each by 7, and so on.

$$\frac{1 \times 6 = 6}{3 \times 6 = 18} \qquad \frac{1 \times 7 = 7}{3 \times 7 = 21}$$

Why does this method of building equivalent fractions work?

- When any number is multiplied by *one*, the number remains unchanged in value.

  ($7 \times 1 = 7$, $8.9 \times 1 = 8.9$, $\frac{1}{2} \times 1 = \frac{1}{2}$, $40 \times 1 = 40$)

- This is also true when *one* appears as a fraction.

  $\frac{1}{1}, \frac{2}{2}, \frac{3}{3}, \frac{4}{4}, \frac{5}{5}, \frac{6}{6}, \frac{7}{7}$...are other ways of writing *one*.

- Multiplying the numerator and denominator each by the same number is the same as multiplying the fraction by *one*.

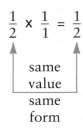

Multiply $\frac{1}{2}$ by one. The *value* and *form* of the fraction remain *unchanged*.

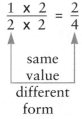

Multiply $\frac{1}{2}$ by other forms of one ($\frac{2}{2}, \frac{3}{3}, \frac{4}{4}, \frac{5}{5}$, etc.). The *value* of the fraction remains unchanged. The *form* of the fraction changes.

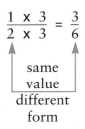

So $\frac{1}{2}, \frac{2}{4}, \frac{3}{6}$, and $\frac{4}{8}$ are equivalent fractions.

It is possible, of course, to make more fractions equivalent to $\frac{1}{2}$. Multiply the fraction $\frac{1}{2}$ by $\frac{5}{5}, \frac{6}{6}, \frac{7}{7}$, and so on.

$$\frac{1 \times 5}{2 \times 5} = \frac{5}{10} \qquad \frac{1 \times 6}{2 \times 6} = \frac{6}{12} \qquad \frac{1 \times 7}{2 \times 7} = \frac{7}{14}$$

Remember that the numerator and denominator are called the terms of the fraction.

Now look at this new set of equivalent fractions.

$$\frac{2}{3} \quad \frac{4}{6} \quad \frac{6}{9} \quad \frac{8}{12} \quad \frac{10}{15} \quad \frac{12}{18} \quad \frac{14}{21}...$$

Even though all of the fractions have equal value, the fraction $\frac{2}{3}$ has the lowest numerator and denominator. It has the **lowest terms** and is said to be in **simplest form**. All of the other fractions have higher numerators and denominators and are said to be in **higher terms** than $\frac{2}{3}$.

Simplifying Fractions to Lowest Terms (Reducing Fractions)

The opposite of building equivalent fractions is reducing (simplifying) fractions to their lowest terms. Multiplication and division are opposite operations.

To build equivalent fractions, the numerator and denominator are each multiplied by the same number. (Any number, that is, except zero.)

To simplify fractions, the numerator and denominator are each divided by the same number. (Any number, that is, except zero.)

$$\frac{5 \times 2}{6 \times 2} = \frac{10}{12} \qquad\qquad \frac{10 \div 2}{12 \div 2} = \frac{5}{6}$$

Building a Fraction VS. Reducing a Fraction

To express a fraction in its lowest terms, divide the numerator and denominator each by the largest number that can be divided into both evenly. When there are no whole numbers, except 1, that will divide the numerator and denominator evenly, the fraction is in lowest terms.

A. Reduce the fraction $\frac{24}{32}$ to lowest terms. Both 24 and 32 can each be divided evenly by 4, but $\frac{6}{8}$ is not lowest terms.

$$\frac{24 \div 4}{32 \div 4} = \frac{6}{8}$$

The numbers 6 and 8 can each be divided evenly by 2, so $\frac{3}{4}$ is lowest terms.

$$\frac{24 \div 4}{32 \div 4} = \frac{6 \div 2}{8 \div 2} = \frac{3}{4}$$

B. Reduce the fraction $\frac{24}{32}$ to lowest terms in one step.
Think of the largest number that will divide evenly into 24 and 32.
1, 2, 3, 4, 6, 8, 12, and 24 will go into 24.
1, 2, 4, 8, 16, and 32 will go into 32.
The largest number that will go into both is 8.

$$\frac{24 \div 8}{32 \div 8} = \frac{3}{4}$$

So $\frac{3}{4}$ has the same value as $\frac{24}{32}$, $\frac{3}{4}$ is in lowest terms.

A fraction can be reduced to its lowest terms in one step if the *largest* number possible is chosen to divide evenly into both the numerator and denominator. Otherwise, it may take more than one step. One way is more efficient, but the result is the same!

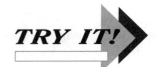

TRY IT!

PRACTICE

Reduce the following fractions to lowest terms. (Simplify.)

> **EXAMPLE**
>
> $$\frac{4 \div 2}{6 \div 2} = \frac{2}{3}$$

1. $\dfrac{15 \div}{20 \div}$ _____ = _____

(The largest number that will divide evenly into both 15 and 20 is 5. $\frac{15}{20} = \frac{3}{4}$)

2. $\dfrac{25 \div}{100 \div}$ _____ = _____

(The largest number that will divide evenly into both 25 and 100 is 25. $\frac{25}{100} = \frac{1}{4}$)

3. $\dfrac{27 \div}{36 \div}$ _____ = _____

(The largest number that will divide evenly into both 27 and 36 is 9. $\frac{27}{36} = \frac{3}{4}$)

Fill in the missing numerator or denominator in the pair of equivalent fractions.

4. $\dfrac{}{3} = \dfrac{16}{24}$

(Look at the fraction that has both terms. Divide each term by the same number. 24 ÷ 8 = 3, so 16 ÷ 8 = 2. $\frac{2}{3} = \frac{16}{24}$)

5. $\dfrac{3}{} = \dfrac{21}{28}$

(Look at the fraction that has both terms. Divide each term by the same number. 21 ÷ 7 = 3, so 28 ÷ 7 = 4. $\frac{3}{4} = \frac{21}{28}$)

6. $\dfrac{5}{6} = \dfrac{35}{}$

(Look at the fraction that has both terms. Multiply each term by the same number. 5 x 7 = 35, so 6 x 7 = 42. $\frac{5}{6} = \frac{35}{42}$)

7. $\dfrac{1}{3} = \dfrac{6}{}$

(Look at the fraction with both terms. Multiply each term by the same number. 1 x 6 = 6, so 3 x 6 = 18. $\frac{1}{3} = \frac{6}{18}$)

ADDITIONAL PRACTICE

Fill in the missing numerator or denominator in each pair of equivalent fractions.

8. $\dfrac{3}{10} = \dfrac{30}{}$ 9. $\dfrac{3}{} = \dfrac{12}{16}$ 10. $\dfrac{2}{3} = \dfrac{}{18}$

11. $\dfrac{}{3} = \dfrac{8}{24}$ 12. $\dfrac{3}{4} = \dfrac{}{24}$ 13. $\dfrac{2}{3} = \dfrac{}{12}$

14. $\dfrac{5}{6} = \dfrac{}{12}$ 15. $\dfrac{3}{4} = \dfrac{}{8}$

Reduce (simplify) each fraction to lowest terms.

16. $\dfrac{10}{15}$ =   17. $\dfrac{5}{25}$ =   18. $\dfrac{6}{9}$ =

19. $\dfrac{10}{12}$ =   20. $\dfrac{27}{36}$ =   21. $\dfrac{16}{32}$ =

Build a set of four more fractions equal to $\frac{4}{5}$.

22. ($\dfrac{4}{5}$, _____, _____, _____, _____)

ON THE JOB

Express all answers in simplest form.

1. On a medical unit, there are 16 patients under age 40 and 18 patients over age 40.
   What fractional part of all the patients are over age 40? _____
   What fractional part of all the patients are under age 40? _____

2. A pharmacist prepared a powder by mixing 6 grams of Compound X and 8 grams of Compound Y.
   What fractional part of the powder is Compound X? _____
   What fractional part of the powder is Compound Y? _____

3. A medicine cup can hold up to 30 milliliters of liquid medication. The cup actually contains 25 milliliters.
   What fractional part of the cup is filled? _____

4. A patient's total intake of fluid in 24 hours was 80 ounces; 30 ounces of the fluid was water.
   What fractional part of the total fluid was water? _____
   What fractional part of the total fluid was liquid other than water? _____

5. One hour is 60 minutes.
   15 minutes represents what fractional part of an hour? _____
   20 minutes represents what fractional part of an hour? _____
   30 minutes represents what fractional part of an hour? _____
   45 minutes represents what fractional part of an hour? _____
   50 minutes represents what fractional part of an hour? _____

PART 5: CONVERTING IMPROPER FRACTIONS TO MIXED NUMBERS AND WHOLE NUMBERS

OBJECTIVE

Change an improper fraction to a mixed number or whole number.

Improper fractions are equal to one or greater than one. Therefore, they can be rewritten in an equivalent form, either as a whole number or a mixed number.

Converting Improper Fractions

An improper fraction has a numerator that is equal to or larger than its denominator. If the numerator is equal to the denominator, the fraction is equal to one whole ($\frac{9}{9} = 1$, $\frac{20}{20} = 1$, $\frac{100}{100} = 1$). If the numerator is larger than the denominator, the fraction can be changed to a mixed number or a whole number ($\frac{9}{4} = 2\frac{1}{4}$, $\frac{8}{4} = 2$).

A mixed number consists of a whole number and a fraction. $2\frac{1}{4}$ is read as "2 and $\frac{1}{4}$" and means $2 + \frac{1}{4}$.

To change an improper fraction to a mixed number or a whole number, divide the numerator by the denominator ($\frac{7}{5} = 7 \div 5$).

A. Change $\frac{15}{6}$ to a mixed number.
   1. 15 equal parts are being considered. It takes 6 equal parts to make 1 whole.
   2. Read the fraction from top to bottom $\frac{15}{6}$ means $15 \div 6$. *Put the numerator "in the house" and divide.*

$$2\frac{3}{6} = 2\frac{1}{2}$$
$$6\overline{)15}$$
$$\underline{12}$$
$$3$$

   3. 2 wholes can be made, which use up 12 of the sixths. 3 of the sixths are left.
   4. Simplify the fraction to the lowest terms.

B. Change $\frac{18}{3}$ to a mixed number (or a whole number).
   1. 18 equal parts are being considered. It takes 3 equal parts to make 1 whole.
   2. Read the fraction from top to bottom. $\frac{18}{3}$ means $18 \div 3$. *Put the numerator "in the house" and divide.*

$$6$$
$$3\overline{)18}$$
$$\underline{18}$$
$$0$$

   3. 6 wholes can be made, which use up 18 of the thirds. There are no thirds left.

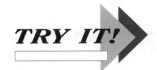
TRY IT!

PRACTICE

Change each improper fraction to its equivalent whole number or improper fraction.

> **EXAMPLES**
>
> $\dfrac{85}{8} = 10\dfrac{5}{8}$ ($85 \div 8 = 10$ wholes and 5 eighths)
>
> $\dfrac{54}{9} = 6$ ($54 \div 9 = 6$ wholes)

1. $\dfrac{70}{8} =$ ($70 \div 8 = 8$ wholes and 6 eighths. $\dfrac{70}{8} = 8\dfrac{6}{8} = 8\dfrac{3}{4}$)

2. $\dfrac{144}{12} =$ ($144 \div 12 = 12$ wholes. $\dfrac{144}{12} = 12$)

3. $\dfrac{39}{9} =$ ($39 \div 9 = 4$ wholes and 3 ninths. $\dfrac{39}{9} = 4\dfrac{3}{9} = 4\dfrac{1}{3}$)

ADDITIONAL PRACTICE

Convert each improper fraction to its mixed number or whole number equivalent in simplified form.

4. $\dfrac{49}{5} =$ 5. $\dfrac{46}{4} =$ 6. $\dfrac{56}{7} =$

7. $\dfrac{54}{8} =$ 8. $\dfrac{47}{5} =$ 9. $\dfrac{22}{8} =$

10. $\dfrac{51}{5} =$ 11. $\dfrac{80}{4} =$ 12. $\dfrac{88}{18} =$

13. $\dfrac{49}{7} =$ 14. $\dfrac{30}{16} =$ 15. $\dfrac{48}{12} =$

16. $\dfrac{22}{6} =$ 17. $\dfrac{22}{4} =$ 18. $\dfrac{37}{3} =$

◆◆◆◆◆◆ **FUN FACTS** ◆◆◆◆◆◆

Two out of three (2/3) American adults wear glasses at some time in their lives.

OBJECTIVE

Change a whole number or mixed number to an improper fraction.

It is necessary to rewrite whole numbers and mixed numbers as their equivalent improper fractions before certain mathematical computations can be performed. This is the opposite of the procedure used in Part 5.

Converting Whole Numbers and Mixed Numbers

To change a whole number to an improper fraction, multiply the whole number times the denominator to find out how many parts are being considered. Keep the denominator.

A. 8 is how many thirds? $\qquad 8 = \dfrac{?}{3}$

Multiply the whole number 8 times the denominator 3 (8 x 3 = 24 thirds).

$$8 = \frac{24}{3}$$

B. 7 is how many fourths? $\qquad 7 = \dfrac{?}{4}$

Multiply the whole number 7 times the denominator 4 (7 x 4 = 28 fourths).

$$7 = \frac{28}{4}$$

C. 9 is how many wholes? $\qquad 9 = \dfrac{?}{1}$

Multiply the whole number 9 times the denominator 1 (9 x 1 = 9 wholes).

$$9 = \frac{9}{1}$$

To change a mixed number to an improper fraction, multiply the whole number times the denominator and then add that product to the numerator. Keep the same denominator.

$$7\frac{2}{3} = \frac{(7 \times 3) + 2}{3} = \frac{23}{3}$$

Even though it is possible to do this procedure in a mechanical way, it is extremely important to understand the "why" behind each step.

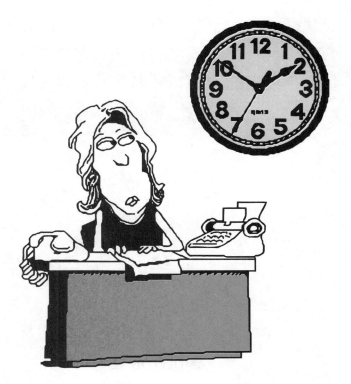

In 1/6 of an hour my boss will be back from his 3-hour lunch. He'll work for 1/4 of an hour and go to the golf course. Such are the burdens of management.

D. Change $7\frac{2}{3}$ to an improper fraction.

1. 7 and $\frac{2}{3}$ means $7 + \frac{2}{3}$. The fractional parts are thirds.
2. Multiply the whole number (7) times the denominator (3) to find out how many thirds are in 7 wholes. 7 x 3 = 21 thirds. $7 = \frac{21}{3}$
3. Add the product of 21 to the numerator 2. Seven wholes have 21 thirds and there are 2 thirds more. 21 thirds + 2 thirds = 23 thirds.
4. Keep the same denominator. The fractional parts were thirds in the beginning and are thirds in the end.

$$7\frac{2}{3} = 7 + \frac{2}{3}$$
$$= \frac{21}{3} + \frac{2}{3} = \frac{23}{3}$$

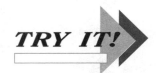

TRY IT!

PRACTICE

Change each mixed number to an improper fraction.

EXAMPLE
$9\frac{3}{7} = \qquad \dfrac{(9 \times 7) + 3}{7} = \dfrac{66}{7}$

1. $10\frac{2}{5} = \qquad \left(\dfrac{(10 \times 5) + 2}{5} = \dfrac{52}{5} \right)$

2. $7\frac{7}{8} = \qquad \left(\dfrac{(7 \times 8) + 7}{8} = \dfrac{63}{8} \right)$

3. $2\frac{8}{9} = \qquad \left(\dfrac{(2 \times 9) + 8}{9} = \dfrac{26}{9} \right)$

4. $7 \quad = \quad \overline{3} \qquad \left(\dfrac{(7 \times 3)}{3} = \dfrac{21}{3} \right)$

ADDITIONAL PRACTICE

Express each mixed number or whole number as its equivalent improper fraction.

5. $7\frac{8}{9} =$ 6. $5\frac{2}{3} =$ 7. $10 \quad =$

8. $5\frac{3}{4} =$ 9. $8\frac{1}{2} =$ 10. $4\frac{7}{8} =$

11. $10\frac{2}{3} =$ 12. $3 \quad =$ 13. $12\frac{1}{4} =$

14. $9\frac{4}{5} =$ 15. $7\frac{3}{4} =$ 16. $15 \quad =$

17. $11\frac{5}{6} =$ 18. $1\frac{7}{8} =$ 19. $6\frac{1}{3} =$

◆◆◆◆◆◆ **FUN FACTS** ◆◆◆◆◆◆

Seven out of 100 men (7/100) suffer from some form of color blindness, while one out of one thousand women (1/1000) have a color-perception deficiency.

PART 7: COMPARING FRACTIONS

OBJECTIVES

1. *Find a common denominator for fractions with unlike denominators.*
2. *Use the symbols (=, >, <) to correctly express comparisons between fractions.*

It is often necessary to know the relative values of numbers. Using several different methods, common fractions may be compared to find the larger or smaller fraction.

Comparing Fractions

When comparing fractions, three symbols are used.

= is equal to	$\frac{7}{8} = \frac{14}{16}$	
> is greater than	$\frac{1}{2} > \frac{3}{14}$	
< is less than	$\frac{3}{10} < \frac{7}{8}$	

Think of the symbols (< and >) as having dots on each side like this:

$$< \qquad >$$

The side with one dot goes next to the smaller number and the side with two dots goes next to the larger number.

$$6 < 8 \qquad \frac{1}{2} > \frac{1}{4}$$

It is not difficult to compare fractions with like denominators, because the size of the pieces is the same.

A. Which fraction is larger, $\frac{5}{8}$ or $\frac{3}{8}$?

5 eighths is greater than 3 eighths.

$$\frac{5}{8} > \frac{3}{8}$$

If the denominators are the same, the fraction with the larger numerator has the greater value.

B. Which fraction is larger, $\frac{3}{4}$ or $\frac{3}{8}$?

In each fraction we are considering or talking about 3 parts. *But the parts are not the same size.* It is necessary to know which parts are larger, the fourths or the eighths. The fewer equal parts in one whole, the larger the parts. If one whole were divided into 4 equal pieces, the pieces would be larger than if the whole were divided into 8 equal parts.

$$\frac{3}{4} > \frac{3}{8}$$

If the numerators are the same, the fraction with the smaller denominator (fewer parts in one whole) has the greater value.

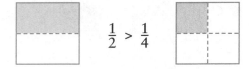

$$\frac{1}{2} > \frac{1}{4}$$

C. Which fraction is larger $\frac{2}{3}$ or $\frac{3}{4}$?

Before it is possible to compare the fractions, they must be rewritten in another form so that they have the same denominators (same size pieces). This is accomplished using skills learned in Part 4: Equivalent Fractions.

To compare $\frac{2}{3}$ and $\frac{3}{4}$, a **common denominator** for both fractions must be found.

A common denominator is a number that can be divided evenly by both denominators. Stated differently, both denominators will go into the common denominator evenly.

Look at the denominators 3 and 4.

3 will go into 3, 6, 9, **12**, and 15...evenly.

4 will go into 4, 8, **12**, and 16...evenly.

What is the lowest number that both 3 and 4 will go into?   (**12**)

12 is the lowest common denominator for the fractions $\frac{2}{3}$ and $\frac{3}{4}$.

Rewrite each fraction as an equivalent fraction using the common denominator.

$$\frac{2 \times 4 = 8}{3 \times 4 = 12} \qquad\qquad \frac{3 \times 3 = 9}{4 \times 3 = 12}$$

Comparing $\frac{2}{3}$ and $\frac{3}{4}$ is the same as comparing $\frac{8}{12}$ and $\frac{9}{12}$.

$$\frac{2}{3} < \frac{3}{4} \qquad \text{because} \qquad \frac{8}{12} < \frac{9}{12}$$

To compare fractions with unlike numerators and denominators, find the lowest common denominator for both fractions. Change each fraction to an equivalent fraction with the lowest common denominator. When both fractions have the same denominator, the fraction with the larger numerator has the larger value.

It is extremely important to be able to compare fractions using the methods presented so far in this section, because the same skills will be used in addition and subtraction of fractions.

However, there is a quick and easy way to compare fractions using cross products.

D. Compare $\frac{2}{3}$ and $\frac{8}{9}$ using cross products.

Multiply the denominator of the first fraction times the numerator of the second fraction (up and over). Write the product *above* the second numerator.

$$\frac{2}{3} \longrightarrow \frac{8}{9}\,^{24}$$

Multiply the denominator of the second fraction times the numerator of the first fraction (up and over). Write the product *above* the first numerator.

$$^{18}\frac{2}{3} \longleftarrow \frac{8}{9}$$

Under the larger product is the larger fraction.

$$^{18}\frac{2}{3} \overset{<}{\times} \frac{8}{9}\,^{24}$$

E. Compare $\frac{5}{8}$ and $\frac{10}{16}$ using cross products.

If the products are equal, the fractions are equal.

$$^{80}\frac{5}{8} \overset{=}{\times} \frac{10}{16}\,^{80}$$

To compare fractions using cross multiplication, write the products of the cross multiplication *above* the fractions. If the products are equal, the fractions are equal. Or, under the larger product is the larger fraction.

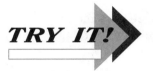

PRACTICE

Find a common denominator for each set of fractions.

EXAMPLE

$\frac{3}{4}, \frac{2}{5}, \frac{1}{10}$ _____   (The lowest common denominator is 20.
4 will go into 4, 8, 12, 16, **20**, 24...
5 will go into 5, 10, 15, **20**, 25...
10 will go into 10, **20**, 30...)

1. $\frac{2}{3}, \frac{3}{5}$ _____   (The lowest common denominator is 15.)

2. $\frac{7}{8}, \frac{1}{4}, \frac{1}{2}$ _____   (The lowest common denominator is 8.)

3. $\frac{8}{9}, \frac{1}{12}$ _____   (The lowest common denominator is 36.)

Compare the fractions using the symbols (less than, greater than, equal to).

4. $\frac{15}{16}$ $\frac{6}{8}$ (> is greater than)

5. $\frac{7}{9}$ $\frac{7}{18}$ (> is greater than)

6. $\frac{3}{7}$ $\frac{5}{6}$ (< is less than)

7. $\frac{8}{9}$ $\frac{32}{36}$ (= is equal to)

ADDITIONAL PRACTICE

Compare the following pairs of fractions using the symbols =, >, or <.

8. $\frac{15}{18}$ $\frac{5}{6}$ 9. $\frac{2}{3}$ $\frac{7}{9}$ 10. $\frac{5}{6}$ $\frac{2}{3}$

11. $\frac{3}{4}$ $\frac{21}{28}$ 12. $\frac{9}{8}$ $\frac{8}{7}$ 13. $\frac{7}{8}$ $\frac{3}{4}$

14. $\frac{5}{12}$ $\frac{3}{4}$ 15. $\frac{3}{10}$ $\frac{12}{40}$ 16. $\frac{4}{10}$ $\frac{5}{9}$

17. $\frac{10}{4}$ $\frac{5}{2}$ 18. $\frac{1}{7}$ $\frac{1}{9}$ 19. $\frac{7}{8}$ $\frac{9}{10}$

20. $\frac{1}{2}$ $\frac{3}{10}$ 21. $\frac{3}{4}$ $\frac{6}{8}$ 22. $\frac{1}{5}$ $\frac{1}{10}$

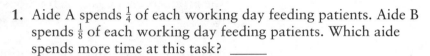

ON THE JOB

1. Aide A spends $\frac{1}{4}$ of each working day feeding patients. Aide B spends $\frac{1}{8}$ of each working day feeding patients. Which aide spends more time at this task? _____

2. One tablet contains $\frac{1}{50}$ grain of medication. Another contains $\frac{1}{100}$ grain. Which is the greater amount of medication? _____

3. One patient's dosage is $\frac{3}{4}$ ounce. Another patient's dosage of the same medication is $\frac{4}{5}$ ounce. Which dosage is greater?

   _____

4. The growth of two babies is compared. Baby X grew $\frac{5}{8}$ inch and Baby Z grew $\frac{7}{16}$ inch. Which baby's length increased more? _____

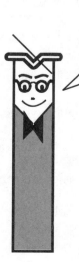

To compare fractions with unlike numerators and denominators, find the lowest common denominator for both fractions. If you're comparing 3/4 oz and 4/5 oz, use 20 as the lowest common denominator.

PART 8: ADDITION AND SUBTRACTION OF FRACTIONS AND MIXED NUMBERS

OBJECTIVES

1. *Add and subtract fractions with like denominators.*
2. *Find a common denominator for fractions having unlike denominators.*
3. *Add and subtract fractions with unlike denominators.*
4. *Add and subtract fractions and mixed numbers.*

When one number is subtracted from another, the answer is called the difference. When numbers are added, the total is called the sum. Fractions must have like denominators before they can be added or subtracted. This means that the pieces being considered must be of the same size. If fractions have unlike denominators, a common denominator must be found before the addition or subtraction can be performed.

Adding and Subtracting Fractions with Like Denominators

To add fractions with a common denominator, add the numerators and write the sum over the common denominator. Express the answer in lowest terms.

To subtract fractions with a common denominator, subtract the numerators and write the difference over the common denominator. Express the answer in lowest terms.

A. Add $\frac{3}{8} + \frac{2}{8} + \frac{5}{8}$.
   1. 3 eighths + 2 eighths + 5 eighths = 10 eighths
   2. $\frac{10}{8}$ is an improper fraction with a value greater than 1.
   3. $10 \div 8 = 1\frac{2}{8}$
   4. Reduce the fractional part. $\frac{2}{8} = \frac{1}{4}$

$$\begin{array}{r} \frac{3}{8} \\ \frac{2}{8} \\ + \frac{5}{8} \\ \hline \frac{10}{8} \end{array} = 1\frac{2}{8} = 1\frac{1}{4}$$

B. Subtract $\frac{1}{8}$ from $\frac{7}{8}$.
   1. 7 eighths minus 1 eighth = 6 eighths
   2. $\frac{6}{8}$ is a proper fraction with a value less than 1.
   3. Reduce the fractional part. $\frac{6}{8} = \frac{3}{4}$

$$\begin{array}{r} \frac{7}{8} \\ - \frac{1}{8} \\ \hline \frac{6}{8} \end{array} = \frac{3}{4}$$

TRY IT!

PRACTICE

Express answers in simplest form.

1. $\frac{1}{5} + \frac{2}{5} + \frac{2}{5} =$ _____ (1 fifth + 2 fifths + 2 fifths = 5 fifths = **1**)

2. $\frac{7}{9} - \frac{1}{9} =$ _____ (7 ninths − 1 ninth = 6 ninths = $\frac{6}{9} = \frac{2}{3}$)

Adding and Subtracting Fractions with Unlike Denominators

Fractions with unlike denominators must first be changed to equivalent fractions with a common denominator. Then the numerators can be added or subtracted, with the resulting sum or difference written over the common denominator. The final answer is expressed in lowest terms.

A. Add $\frac{2}{3} + \frac{3}{4} + \frac{1}{6}$.

1. Thirds, fourths, and sixths are not the same size pieces. A common denominator is needed. What is the lowest number that 3, 4, and 6 will all go into evenly?

   3 will go into 3, 6, 9, **12**, 15...evenly.
   4 will go into 4, 8, **12**, 16...evenly.
   6 will go into 6, **12**, 18...evenly.
   3, 4, and 6 will all go into 12 evenly.

   12 is the common denominator.

2. Make equivalent fractions for $\frac{2}{3}$, $\frac{3}{4}$, and $\frac{1}{6}$ using the common denominator of 12. Now the problem is restated in equal form.

   8 twelfths + 9 twelfths + 2 twelfths

$$\frac{2}{3} = \frac{8}{12}$$
$$\frac{3}{4} = \frac{9}{12}$$
$$+\frac{1}{6} = \frac{2}{12}$$
$$\overline{\qquad\qquad} $$
$$\frac{19}{12} = 1\frac{7}{12}$$

3. Add the numerators of the like fractions and place the sum (19) over the common denominator (12).

$$\frac{19}{12} = 19 \div 12 = 1\frac{7}{12}$$

B. Subtract $\frac{9}{16}$ from $\frac{3}{4}$.

1. Fourths and sixteenths are not the same size pieces. A common denominator is needed. What is the lowest number that 4 and 16 will both go into evenly?

   4 will go into 4, 8, 12, **16**, 20 evenly.
   16 will go into **16**, 32 evenly.
   4 and 16 will both go into 16 evenly.

   16 is the lowest common denominator.

2. Make equivalent fractions for $\frac{3}{4}$ and $\frac{9}{16}$ using the common denominator of 16. Now the problem is restated in an equal form. 12 sixteenths – 9 sixteenths.

$$\frac{3}{4} = \frac{12}{16}$$
$$-\frac{9}{16} = \frac{9}{16}$$
$$\overline{\qquad\qquad}$$
$$\frac{3}{16}$$

3. Subtract the numerators and place the difference over the common denominator.

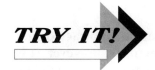

TRY IT!

PRACTICE

Express answers in simplest form.

ANSWERS

1. $\frac{3}{8} + \frac{1}{2} + \frac{3}{4} =$

$$
\begin{aligned}
\mathbf{1.} \quad \frac{3}{8} &= \frac{3}{8} \\
\frac{1}{2} &= \frac{4}{8} \\
+ \frac{3}{4} &= \frac{6}{8} \\
\hline
\frac{13}{8} &= 1\frac{5}{8}
\end{aligned}
$$

2. $\frac{9}{9} - \frac{2}{3} =$

$$
\begin{aligned}
\mathbf{2.} \quad \frac{9}{9} &= \frac{9}{9} \\
- \frac{2}{3} &= \frac{6}{9} \\
\hline
\frac{3}{9} &= \frac{1}{3}
\end{aligned}
$$

Adding Mixed Numbers

When adding mixed numbers, the fractional parts are added first. This sum is added to the sum of the whole numbers. The final answer is written in simplest form.

$$3\frac{3}{4} + 4\frac{5}{6} =$$

1. Express the fractions $\frac{3}{4}$ and $\frac{5}{6}$ in equivalent forms using the common denominator. 4 and 6 will both divide evenly into 12.
2. Add the fractions first.
3. Then add the whole numbers.
4. Express the answer in simplest form.

$$
\begin{aligned}
3\frac{3}{4} &= 3\frac{9}{12} \\
+ 4\frac{5}{6} &= 4\frac{10}{12} \\
\hline
7\frac{19}{12} &= 8\frac{7}{12}
\end{aligned}
$$

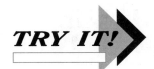

TRY IT!

PRACTICE

Express answers in simplest form.

1. $3\frac{7}{8} + 5\frac{5}{8} = \underline{\hspace{1cm}}$

2. $7\frac{9}{10} + 3\frac{4}{5} = \underline{\hspace{1cm}}$

ANSWERS

1. $3\frac{7}{8}$
   $+ 5\frac{5}{8}$
   $\overline{}$
   $8\frac{12}{8} = 8 + 1\frac{4}{8} = 9\frac{4}{8} = 9\frac{1}{2}$

2. $7\frac{9}{10} = 7\frac{9}{10}$
   $+ 3\frac{4}{5} = 3\frac{8}{10}$
   $\overline{}$
   $10\frac{17}{10} = 10 + 1\frac{7}{10} = 11\frac{7}{10}$

Subtracting Mixed Numbers

When subtracting mixed numbers, the fractions are subtracted first and then the whole numbers are subtracted. Sometimes, however, it is necessary to "borrow" (or regroup) before subtracting, just as is done with whole numbers. The mixed numbers or whole numbers are expressed in another equivalent form before subtracting.

Examples of regrouping ("borrowing").

1. 1 is "borrowed" from the whole number and written as a fraction.
$6 = 5\frac{8}{8}$
$8 = 7\frac{3}{3}$

2. 1 is "borrowed" from the whole number and added to the fractional part of the number.
$2\frac{4}{12} = 1\frac{16}{12}$
$6\frac{3}{8} = 5\frac{11}{8}$

The following examples illustrate four different situations.

A. Subtract $4\frac{3}{4}$ from $6\frac{7}{8}$. $(6\frac{7}{8} - 4\frac{3}{4})$

1. Rewrite the problem, expressing the fractions with a common denominator.
2. Try to subtract the fractions 7 eighths – 6 eighths = 1 eighth
3. Subtract the whole numbers. $6 - 4 = 2$
4. Simplify the answer, if possible.

$$
\begin{array}{rcl}
6\frac{7}{8} &=& 6\frac{7}{8} \\
- 4\frac{3}{4} &=& 4\frac{6}{8} \\
\hline
&& 2\frac{1}{8}
\end{array}
$$

B. Subtract $1\frac{3}{4}$ from $2\frac{1}{3}$. $(2\frac{1}{3} - 1\frac{3}{4})$

1. Rewrite the problem, expressing the fractions with a common denominator.
2. Try to subtract the fractions. 4 twelfths – 9 twelfths = WHAT??? If there are only 4 parts, it seems impossible to take away 9 parts!
3. Borrow $\frac{12}{12}$ from the whole number. (That is the same as borrowing 1.) Add the $\frac{12}{12}$ to the $\frac{4}{12}$ that are already there. Now there are $\frac{16}{12}$ in the fractional part and only 1 in the whole number.
4. Now try to subtract the fractions. 16 twelfths – 9 twelfths = 7 twelfths
5. Subtract the whole numbers. $1 - 1 = 0$
6. Simplify the answer, if possible.

$$
\begin{array}{rclcl}
2\frac{1}{3} &=& 2\frac{4}{12} \\
- 1\frac{3}{4} &=& 1\frac{9}{12} \\
\hline
2\frac{1}{3} &=& 2\frac{4}{12} &=& 1\frac{16}{12} \\
- 1\frac{3}{4} &=& 1\frac{9}{12} &=& 1\frac{9}{12} \\
\hline
&&&& \frac{7}{12}
\end{array}
$$

C. Subtract $\frac{7}{8}$ from 6. $(6 - \frac{7}{8})$

1. Try to subtract the fractions. No eighths – 7 eighths = WHAT???
2. 6 must be rewritten in an equivalent form that is useful in solving the problem. Since the problem deals with *eighths*, 1 is borrowed from the whole number as $\frac{8}{8}$. $(6 = 5\frac{8}{8})$
3. Now try to subtract the fractions. 8 eighths – 7 eighths = 1 eighth
4. Subtract the whole numbers. $5 - 0 = 5$

$$
\begin{array}{rl}
6 & = 5\frac{8}{8} \\
-\ \frac{7}{8} & = \ \ \frac{7}{8} \\
\hline
& \ \ 5\frac{1}{8}
\end{array}
$$

D. Subtract 6 from $8\frac{3}{4}$. $(8\frac{3}{4} - 6)$

1. Try to subtract the fractions. 3 fourths – 0 fourths = 3 fourths
2. Subtract the whole numbers. $8 - 6 = 2$
3. Simplify the answer, if possible.

$$
\begin{array}{r}
8\frac{3}{4} \\
-\ 6 \\
\hline
2\frac{3}{4}
\end{array}
$$

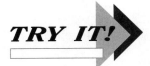

PRACTICE

Regroup (borrow) if necessary. Express answers in simplest form.

1. $7\frac{7}{8} - \frac{3}{4} =$ _____

2. $11 - 3\frac{2}{8} =$ _____

3. $6\frac{1}{3} - 2\frac{3}{4} =$ _____

ANSWERS

1.
$$
\begin{array}{rl}
7\frac{7}{8} & = 7\frac{7}{8} \\
-\ \frac{3}{4} & = \ \ \frac{6}{8} \\
\hline
& \ \ 7\frac{1}{8}
\end{array}
$$

2.
$$
\begin{array}{rl}
11 & = 10\frac{8}{8} \\
-\ 3\frac{2}{8} & = \ \ 3\frac{2}{8} \\
\hline
& \ \ 7\frac{6}{8} = 7\frac{3}{4}
\end{array}
$$

3.
$$
\begin{array}{rll}
6\frac{1}{3} & = 6\frac{4}{12} & = 5\frac{16}{12} \\
-2\frac{3}{4} & = 2\frac{9}{12} & = 2\frac{9}{12} \\
\hline
& & \ \ 3\frac{7}{12}
\end{array}
$$

ADDITIONAL PRACTICE

Add or subtract the common fractions as designated. Express the answers in lowest terms.

4. $\frac{11}{16} - \frac{5}{16} =$ 5. $\frac{7}{8} - \frac{1}{5} =$ 6. $\frac{5}{6} - \frac{1}{2} =$

7. $\frac{7}{10} - \frac{3}{10} =$ 8. $\frac{2}{3} + \frac{3}{4} =$ 9. $\frac{3}{4} - \frac{5}{12} =$

10. $\frac{2}{5} + \frac{1}{6} =$ 11. $\frac{11}{16} - \frac{9}{20} =$ 12. $\frac{3}{4} - \frac{2}{5} =$

13. $\frac{2}{3} - \frac{7}{16} =$

Add or subtract the mixed numbers and fractions as designated. Express the answers in lowest terms.

14. $7\frac{3}{4} + 6 =$ 15. $8\frac{1}{3} - 1\frac{5}{6} =$ 16. $10\frac{7}{10} + 8\frac{4}{5} =$

17. $8\frac{3}{8} - \frac{7}{8} =$ 18. $4\frac{3}{10} + 7\frac{7}{10} =$ 19. $5 - 2\frac{5}{8} =$

20. $8\frac{2}{3} - 7 =$ 21. $8\frac{4}{5} - 2\frac{1}{2} =$ 22. $6\frac{3}{4} + 6\frac{5}{6} =$

23. $3\frac{3}{10} + 4\frac{9}{16} =$

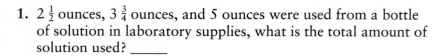

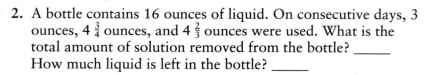

ON THE JOB

• • • • • • • • • • •

1. $2\frac{1}{2}$ ounces, $3\frac{3}{4}$ ounces, and 5 ounces were used from a bottle of solution in laboratory supplies, what is the total amount of solution used? _____

2. A bottle contains 16 ounces of liquid. On consecutive days, 3 ounces, $4\frac{3}{4}$ ounces, and $4\frac{2}{3}$ ounces were used. What is the total amount of solution removed from the bottle? _____ How much liquid is left in the bottle? _____

3. Two months ago Patient A weighed $124\frac{1}{4}$ pounds. Now the patient weighs $115\frac{3}{4}$ pounds. How many pounds did Patient A lose? _____

4. If normal body temperature is $98\frac{3}{5}$ degrees Fahrenheit, how many degrees above normal is $101\frac{1}{2}$ degrees? _____

5. A patient needs to drink $4\frac{1}{2}$ pints of liquid in one day. If $3\frac{2}{3}$ pints have been consumed, how much more liquid is needed?

_____

PART 9: MULTIPLICATION OF FRACTIONS AND MIXED NUMBERS

OBJECTIVE

Multiply fractions and mixed numbers.

When numbers are multiplied, the answer is called the product. The numbers that are multiplied are called factors (Factor x Factor = Product).

Multiplication of Fractions and Mixed Numbers

Before multiplying fractions and mixed numbers, the factors must all be expressed as fractions first. Mixed numbers are written as improper fractions ($6\frac{1}{2} = \frac{13}{2}$). Whole numbers are written as fractions by putting the whole number over the denominator 1 ($5 = \frac{5}{1}$).

$$6\frac{1}{2} \times 5 \times \frac{3}{4} = \frac{13}{2} \times \frac{5}{1} \times \frac{3}{4}$$

When all of the factors have been expressed as fractions, multiply the numerators first. Then multiply the denominators. Simplify the answer if necessary. Change improper fractions to mixed numbers. Reduce fractions to lowest terms.

$$6\frac{1}{2} \times 5 \times \frac{3}{4} = \frac{13}{2} \times \frac{5}{1} \times \frac{3}{4} = \frac{195}{8} = 24\frac{3}{8}$$

A. Multiply $\frac{1}{2} \times \frac{2}{3}$.
   1. $\frac{1}{2} \times \frac{2}{3}$ means $\frac{1}{2}$ of $\frac{2}{3}$.
   2. Look at the amount $\frac{2}{3}$.
   3. Shade $\frac{1}{2}$ of it.

   4. Multiply the numerators.
   5. Multiply the denominators. $\frac{1}{2} \times \frac{2}{3} = \frac{2}{6} = \frac{1}{3}$
   6. Simplify if necessary.

B. Multiply $3 \times \frac{2}{3}$.
   1. $3 \times \frac{2}{3}$ means 3 of the $\frac{2}{3}$'s.
   2. Look at 3 of the $\frac{2}{3}$'s. How many thirds are there altogether? 6 thirds.

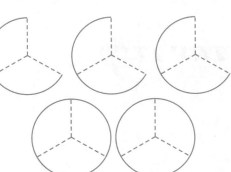

   3. Rearrange the 6 thirds.

   4. Express 3 as a fraction. $3 = \frac{3}{1}$.
   5. Multiply numerator x numerator.
   6. Multiply denominator x denominator. $\frac{3}{1} \times \frac{2}{3} = \frac{6}{3} = \frac{2}{1} = 2$
   7. Simplify the answer, if necessary.

C. Multiply $\frac{15}{28} \times \frac{7}{30}$.
1. Multiply numerator × numerator.
2. Multiply denominator × denominator.
3. Reduce the fraction to lowest terms. (Divide the numerator and denominator each by the largest number that will go into both evenly. That is, 105.)

$$\frac{15}{28} \times \frac{7}{30} = \frac{105}{840} + \frac{105}{105} = \frac{1}{8}$$

4. THIS IS TOO MUCH WORK! Who would think of 105, anyway?

To make multiplication of fractions easier, there is a short-cut! The short-cut is called cancellation. It is like reducing *before* you multiply, instead of reducing the answer *after* you have multiplied. WARNING: Always check the final answer to make sure it is in lowest terms, even if cancellation has been used.

D. Again. Multiply $\frac{15}{28} \times \frac{7}{30}$.
1. Notice that the numerator in $\frac{15}{28}$ and the denominator in $\frac{7}{30}$ can each be divided by 15.

$$\frac{\overset{1}{\cancel{15}}}{28} \times \frac{7}{\underset{2}{\cancel{30}}}$$

2. Notice that the numerator in $\frac{7}{30}$ and the denominator in $\frac{15}{28}$ can each be divided by 7.

$$\frac{\overset{1}{\cancel{15}}}{\underset{4}{\cancel{28}}} \times \frac{\overset{1}{\cancel{7}}}{\underset{2}{\cancel{30}}}$$

3. Now multiply numerator × numerator.
4. Multiply denominator × denominator.

$$\frac{1}{4} \times \frac{1}{2} = \frac{1}{8}$$

5. Simplify the answer if necessary.
6. ISN'T THIS EASIER?

E. Multiply $3 \times \frac{2}{9} \times \frac{9}{10}$.

$$\frac{3}{1} \times \frac{\overset{1}{\cancel{2}}}{\underset{1}{\cancel{9}}} \times \frac{\overset{1}{\cancel{9}}}{\underset{5}{\cancel{10}}} = \frac{3}{5}$$

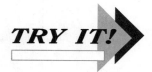
TRY IT!

PRACTICE

Remember to write whole numbers and mixed numbers as improper fractions before multiplying. Use the cancellation short-cut if possible. Simplify the answers.

1. $\frac{3}{9} \times \frac{9}{10} \times 4 =$

2. $\frac{18}{35} \times 7\frac{7}{9} =$

ANSWERS

1. $\frac{3}{9} \times \frac{\overset{1}{\cancel{9}}}{\underset{5}{\cancel{10}}} \times \frac{\overset{2}{\cancel{4}}}{1} = \frac{6}{5} = 1\frac{1}{5}$

2. $\frac{\overset{2}{\cancel{18}}}{\underset{1}{\cancel{35}}} \times \frac{\overset{2}{\cancel{70}}}{\underset{1}{\cancel{9}}} = \frac{4}{1} = 4$

ADDITIONAL PRACTICE

Change all mixed numbers and whole numbers to improper fractions before multiplying. Use the cancellation short-cut whenever possible. Simplify the answers.

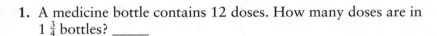

3. $\frac{5}{6} \times 8 =$ 4. $\frac{2}{3} \times \frac{6}{7} =$ 5. $4\frac{4}{5} \times \frac{5}{6} =$

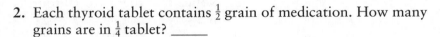

6. $2\frac{1}{2} \times 7 =$ 7. $\frac{1}{2} \times \frac{2}{5} =$ 8. $2 \times \frac{3}{4} =$

9. $5 \times 3\frac{1}{3} =$ 10. $3\frac{3}{8} \times 2\frac{2}{3} =$ 11. $6\frac{7}{8} \times 1 =$

12. $2\frac{5}{8} \times 2\frac{1}{4} =$

ON THE JOB

1. A medicine bottle contains 12 doses. How many doses are in $1\frac{3}{4}$ bottles? _____

2. Each thyroid tablet contains $\frac{1}{2}$ grain of medication. How many grains are in $\frac{1}{4}$ tablet? _____

3. One tablet contains 250 milligrams of medication. How many milligrams are in $2\frac{3}{4}$ tablets? _____

4. A medicine cup can hold up to 30 cc (cubic centimeters) of liquid. If $\frac{3}{5}$ of the cup is full, how many cubic centimeters of liquid are in the cup? _____

PART 10: DIVISION OF FRACTIONS AND MIXED NUMBERS

OBJECTIVES

1. *Find the reciprocal of proper fractions, mixed numbers, and whole numbers.*
2. *Divide fractions and mixed numbers.*

When one number is divided by another, the answer is called the quotient (dividend ÷ divisor = quotient or dividend/divisor = quotient). It will be shown in this part that dividing by a number is the same as multiplying by its reciprocal.

Dividing Fractions and Mixed Numbers

Think of division problems in words.

A. Divide $2\frac{1}{2}$ by $\frac{1}{4}$.

1. $2\frac{1}{2} \div \frac{1}{4}$ means "How many fourths are in $2\frac{1}{2}$?"
2. Look at $2\frac{1}{2}$.
3. Notice that there are 10 fourths in $2\frac{1}{2}$.
4. $2\frac{1}{2} \div \frac{1}{4} = \frac{5}{2} \div \frac{1}{4} = 10$
5. It is easy to observe that there are 10 fourths in $2\frac{1}{2}$ but the mathematical equation may not make sense.

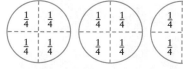

Division involves the use of a reciprocal (or inverse). The reciprocal of a fraction is its "flip." Change mixed numbers and whole numbers to their equivalent improper fractions first. Then find the reciprocal of the divisor by inverting (flipping) it.

Fraction	Reciprocal (Invert the fraction)
$\frac{7}{8}$	$\frac{8}{7}$
$3\frac{1}{4} = \frac{13}{4}$	$\frac{4}{13}$
$6 = \frac{6}{1}$	$\frac{1}{6}$

Remember, dividing by a number is the same as multiplying by its reciprocal. So dividing by 10 is the same as multiplying by $\frac{1}{10}$. Or dividing by 7 is the same as multiplying by $\frac{1}{7}$.

B. Divide $\frac{3}{4}$ by $\frac{1}{4}$ ($\frac{3}{4} \div \frac{1}{4}$).

1. How many fourths are in 3 fourths?   3
2. Dividing by a fraction is the same as multiplying times its reciprocal.

$$\frac{3}{4} \div \frac{1}{4} = \frac{3}{4} \times \frac{4}{1} = \frac{12}{4} = \frac{3}{1} = 3$$

Before dividing mixed numbers and fractions, the problem must be expressed in the form of all fractions. Whole numbers and mixed numbers are written as improper fractions ($8 = \frac{8}{1}$, $4\frac{1}{5} = \frac{21}{5}$).

C. Divide 8 by $4\frac{1}{5}$.

$$8 \div 4\frac{1}{5} = \frac{8}{1} \div \frac{21}{5} =$$

Remember that dividing by a fraction is the same as multiplying by its reciprocal. Invert the *second* fraction. Multiply the first fraction times *the reciprocal of the second fraction*. Use cancellation when multiplying, if possible. Simplify all final answers.

$$8 \div 4\frac{1}{5} = \frac{8}{1} \div \frac{21}{5} = \frac{8}{1} \times \frac{5}{21} = \frac{40}{21} = 1\frac{19}{21}$$

Original Division Problem	Division Problem As Fractions	Expressed As Multiplication Using the Reciprocal. Use cancellation, if possible. Multiply	Simplify

D.

$$2\frac{1}{3} \div 7 = \qquad \frac{7}{3} \div \frac{7}{1} = \qquad \frac{\overset{1}{7}}{3} \times \frac{1}{\underset{1}{7}} = \frac{1}{3}$$

E.

$$5\frac{5}{8} \div 2\frac{1}{2} = \qquad \frac{45}{8} \div \frac{5}{2} = \qquad \frac{\overset{9}{45}}{\underset{4}{8}} \times \frac{\overset{1}{2}}{\underset{1}{5}} = \qquad\qquad \frac{9}{4} = 2\frac{1}{4}$$

Complex Fractions

A fraction where one or both terms is a fraction is called a complex fraction. The fraction bar separating the numerator and denominator is longer to avoid confusion. Think of the fraction bar separating the fractions as "divided by," as was done before.

A. $\dfrac{\frac{1}{2}}{3} = \frac{1}{2} \div \frac{3}{1} = \frac{1}{2} \times \frac{1}{3} = \frac{1}{6}$

B. $\dfrac{6}{\frac{3}{4}} = \frac{6}{1} \div \frac{3}{4} = \frac{6}{1} \times \frac{4}{3} = \frac{8}{1} = 8$

C. $\dfrac{\frac{3}{4}}{\frac{1}{2}} = \frac{3}{4} \div \frac{1}{2} = \frac{3}{4} \times \frac{2}{1} = \frac{3}{2} = 1\frac{1}{2}$

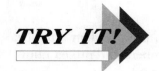

PRACTICE

Write the reciprocal for each number. (Change whole numbers and mixed numbers to improper fractions first.)

1. $\frac{8}{9}$ reciprocal _____ $(\frac{9}{8})$

2. $6\frac{3}{4}$ reciprocal _____ $(6\frac{3}{4} = \frac{27}{4}$ reciprocal $\frac{4}{27})$

3. 10 reciprocal _____ $(10 = \frac{10}{1}$ reciprocal $\frac{1}{10})$

Change all whole numbers and mixed numbers to improper fractions before dividing.

4. $25 \div 8\frac{1}{3} = $ _____ $(25 \div 8\frac{1}{3} = \frac{25}{1} \div \frac{25}{3} = \frac{25}{1} \times \frac{3}{25} = \frac{3}{1} = 3)$

5. $\frac{3}{4} \div 12\frac{1}{2} = $ _____ $(\frac{3}{4} \div 12\frac{1}{2} = \frac{3}{4} \div \frac{25}{2} = \frac{3}{4} \times \frac{2}{25} = \frac{3}{50})$

6. $36\frac{1}{4} \div 3\frac{3}{4} = $ _____ $(36\frac{1}{4} \div 3\frac{3}{4} = \frac{145}{4} \div \frac{15}{4} = \frac{145}{4} \times \frac{4}{15} = \frac{29}{3} = 9\frac{2}{3})$

7. $\dfrac{\frac{3}{8}}{\frac{3}{4}} = $ _____ $(\frac{3}{8} \div \frac{3}{4} = \frac{3}{8} \times \frac{4}{3} = \frac{1}{2})$

ADDITIONAL PRACTICE

Change all mixed numbers and whole numbers to improper fractions before dividing. Use the cancellation short-cut whenever possible. Simplify the answers.

8. $\frac{3}{4} \div \frac{3}{5}$

9. $5\frac{1}{4} \div 5\frac{1}{4}$

10. $1\frac{1}{6} \div 9\frac{1}{3}$

11. $7\frac{3}{4} \div 3$

12. $2\frac{1}{2} \div \frac{5}{6}$

13. $5 \div \frac{3}{4}$

14. $2\frac{3}{16} \div 1\frac{1}{4}$

15. $\frac{7}{8} \div \frac{5}{12}$

16. $2\frac{1}{2} \div \frac{3}{4}$

17. $\frac{1}{2} \div 10$

18. $6\frac{3}{5} \div 1\frac{1}{10}$

19. $\frac{5}{6} \div \frac{2}{5}$

20. $10 \div \frac{2}{5}$

21. $\frac{8}{9} \div 2\frac{2}{3}$

22. $4 \div 1\frac{1}{3}$

1. A bottle of medication contains 6 ounces.
   A. How many $\frac{3}{4}$ ounce doses are in the 6 ounce bottle? _____
   B. How many $1\frac{1}{4}$ ounce doses are in the 6 ounce bottle? _____

2. How many $\frac{2}{3}$ hour time periods are in $6\frac{1}{2}$ hours? _____

3. There are 15 milligrams of medication left in the bottle. How many *full* $2\frac{1}{4}$ milligram doses can be administered from the remaining medication? _____

4. The prescribed dosage of a medication is $5\frac{1}{4}$ grains. Each tablet contains $1\frac{3}{4}$ grains. How many tablets are needed to administer the prescribed dosage? _____

5. A medicine bottle contains 15 doses.
   A. How many bottles are necessary for 20 doses? _____
   B. How many bottles are necessary for 5 doses? _____

◆◆◆◆◆ FUN FACTS ◆◆◆◆◆

Only four poems out of more than nine hundred (4/900) written by Emily Dickinson were published in her lifetime.

EXERCISES

Write a common fraction (proper or improper) equivalent to each phrase.

1. 8 out of a total of 11 _____

2. 17 divided by 9 _____

3. 7 of the thirds _____

4. 9 wholes _____

5. 5 out of a total of 6 _____

6. 7 ÷ 8 _____

7. 5 of the halves _____

8. 1 whole _____

9. 9 out of a total of 10 _____

Identify each fraction as proper (P) or improper (I). Then tell if the fraction is =1, >1, or <1.

10. $\frac{3}{8}$ _____ _____

11. $\frac{100}{100}$ _____ _____

12. $\frac{10}{7}$ _____ _____

13. $\frac{3}{4}$ _____ _____

14. $\frac{5}{5}$ _____ _____

15. $\frac{2}{3}$ _____ _____

16. $\frac{7}{1}$ _____ _____

17. $\frac{7}{7}$ _____ _____

18. $\frac{1}{1}$ _____ _____

19. $\frac{1}{4}$ _____ _____

Fill in the appropriate numerator or denominator in the equivalent fraction pairs.

20. $\frac{}{12}$ = $\frac{3}{4}$

21. $\frac{1}{2}$ = $\frac{}{50}$

22. $\frac{3}{}$ = $\frac{24}{64}$

23. $\frac{12}{36}$ = $\frac{2}{}$

24. $\frac{75}{100}$ = $\frac{}{4}$

Reduce each fraction to lowest terms.

25. $\frac{36}{42}$ _____

26. $\frac{30}{100}$ _____

27. $\frac{24}{32}$ _____

28. $\frac{12}{18}$ _____

29. $\frac{8}{24}$ _____

30. $\frac{7}{14}$ _____

Change each improper fraction to its equivalent whole number or mixed number in simplest form.

31. $\frac{300}{75}$ _____

32. $\frac{10}{8}$ _____

33. $\frac{100}{100}$ _____

34. $\frac{16}{5}$ _____

35. $\frac{24}{7}$ _____

36. $\frac{30}{4}$ _____

Change each whole or mixed number to its equivalent improper fraction.

37. $12 = \dfrac{}{3}$ **38.** $9\dfrac{3}{4} = $ ____   **39.** $10\dfrac{3}{8} = $ ____

40. $6\dfrac{4}{5} = $ ____   **41.** $2\dfrac{8}{9} = $ ____   **42.** $5 = \dfrac{}{7}$

Compare the fractions using the symbols =, >, or <.

43. $\dfrac{7}{9}$ ___ $\dfrac{3}{18}$ **44.** $\dfrac{1}{15}$ ___ $\dfrac{1}{9}$ **45.** $\dfrac{7}{10}$ ___ $\dfrac{4}{10}$

46. $\dfrac{50}{100}$ ___ $\dfrac{1}{2}$ **47.** $\dfrac{2}{3}$ ___ $\dfrac{15}{20}$ **48.** $\dfrac{7}{8}$ ___ $\dfrac{8}{9}$

Add. Express the sum in lowest terms.

49. $3\dfrac{3}{4} + \dfrac{7}{8} + \dfrac{1}{2} = $ ____   **50.** $\dfrac{1}{2} + \dfrac{3}{10} + \dfrac{4}{5} = $ ____

51. $3\dfrac{3}{10} + 7\dfrac{1}{10} = $ ____   **52.** $\dfrac{5}{6} + \dfrac{1}{6} + \dfrac{1}{6} = $ ____

53. $8\dfrac{2}{3} + 6\dfrac{1}{2} + 4\dfrac{5}{8} = $ ____   **54.** $\dfrac{3}{4} + \dfrac{3}{4} = $ ____

Subtract. Express the difference in lowest terms.

55. $6 - 3\dfrac{3}{4} = $ ____   **56.** $4\dfrac{3}{5} - 2\dfrac{1}{3} = $ ____

57. $\dfrac{5}{8} - \dfrac{1}{8} = $ ____   **58.** $10 - \dfrac{4}{5} = $ ____

59. $\dfrac{7}{8} - \dfrac{1}{5} = $ ____   **60.** $27\dfrac{3}{5} - 14\dfrac{3}{5} = $ ____

Multiply. Express the product in lowest terms.

61. $\dfrac{1}{5} \times \dfrac{2}{3} = $ ____   **62.** $\dfrac{3}{4} \times \dfrac{8}{15} = $ ____

63. $\dfrac{7}{8} \times 8 = $ ____   **64.** $\dfrac{3}{4} \times 2 = $ ____

65. $4 \times \dfrac{7}{8} = $ ____   **66.** $5 \times 1\dfrac{5}{6} = $ ____

Divide. Express the quotient in lowest terms.

67. $\dfrac{3}{4} \div 6 = $ ____   **68.** $4\dfrac{1}{2} \div 9 = $ ____

69. $\dfrac{1}{3} \div \dfrac{3}{4} = $ ____   **70.** $4 \div 5\dfrac{1}{3} = $ ____

71. $2\dfrac{1}{2} \div \dfrac{5}{6} = $ ____   **72.** $17\dfrac{1}{2} \div 17\dfrac{1}{2} = $ ____

73. $9\dfrac{1}{3} \div 3\dfrac{1}{7} = $ ____

1. A pharmacist prepares a mixture containing 5 grams of compound A and 7 grams of compound B.
   What fractional part of the whole mixture is compound A? _____
   What fractional part of the whole mixture is compound B? _____

2. One patient's dosage is $\frac{3}{4}$ ounce. Another patient's dosage of the same medication is $\frac{7}{8}$ ounce. Which dosage is greater? _____

3. The following doses of medication were administered: $1\frac{7}{8}$ ounces, $1\frac{3}{4}$ ounces, and $1\frac{1}{2}$ ounces. What is the total number of ounces given? _____

4. The dosage to be given in one day is 8 grains; $4\frac{3}{4}$ grains have been administered. How many grains are left to be given? _____

5. A tablet contains 500 milligrams of Tylenol. How many milligrams are in $6\frac{3}{4}$ tablets? _____

6. How many $1\frac{1}{4}$ ounce doses are in an $8\frac{3}{4}$ ounce bottle? _____

7. A medicine cup holds 30 milliliters of liquid. How many medicine cups are necessary to administer 45 milliliters of medication? _____

8. If $2\frac{1}{2}$ tablets were administered with breakfast, 2 tablets with lunch, and $1\frac{3}{4}$ tablets with dinner, how many tablets were given altogether? _____

9. A tablet contains 300 milligrams of medication. How many milligrams are contained in $\frac{1}{8}$ tablet? _____

10. The surgeon requested 10 pints of dextrose solution for surgery; $6\frac{1}{8}$ pints remain after surgery. How many pints were used? _____

11. Which is the greater amount of time, $\frac{7}{12}$ hour or $\frac{3}{4}$ hour? _____

12. A medicine cup can hold up to 30 cc (cubic centimeters) of medication. The cup actually contains 18 cc (cubic centimeters) of liquid. What fractional part of the cup is filled? _____

13. One teaspoonful of children's Tylenol contains 160 milligrams of Tylenol. Then 45 milligrams is what fractional part of that dose? _____

14. There are 10 males and 14 females in the mathematics class. What fractional part of the whole class are the females? _____ What fractional part of the whole class are males? _____

15. Baby A grew $\frac{3}{8}$ inch. Baby B grew $\frac{5}{16}$ inch. Which baby's length increased more? _____

16. The dosage to be given in one day is 8 ounces; $2\frac{2}{3}$ ounces and $3\frac{5}{16}$ ounces have been administered. How much medication remains to be administered? _____

17. An audit revealed that $\frac{2}{7}$ of the 49 patients had been prescribed a mood elevator.
    How many patients were given a mood elevator? _____
    How many patients were *not* given a mood elevator? _____

18. There are $7\frac{3}{4}$ ounces of solution in a container.
    How many ounces is $\frac{1}{4}$ of that solution? _____
    How many ounces is $\frac{3}{4}$ of that solution? _____

19. How many hours elapsed if $\frac{2}{3}$ of an hour was spent in therapy, $1\frac{5}{12}$ hours in recreation, and $2\frac{1}{4}$ hours in testing? _____

20. How many $1\frac{3}{20}$ hour time periods are in $7\frac{1}{2}$ hours? _____

2 *Decimals*

PART 1: INTRODUCTION TO DECIMAL FRACTIONS AND MIXED DECIMALS

OBJECTIVES

1. *Read decimal numbers.*
2. *Write the common fraction or mixed number equivalent of a decimal number.*
3. *Write the decimal equivalent of a mixed number or common fraction (with denominators of 10, 100, 1000, etc.).*

The decimal system is based on the number ten. A decimal point separates the wholes from the fractional parts. This section addresses both decimal fractions and mixed decimals.

Decimal Fractions

Decimal fractions represent common fractions that have denominators of 10, 100, 1000, or some power of 10. In a decimal fraction, the position of a number relative to the decimal point indicates value. To the left of the decimal point are whole numbers and to the right of the decimal point are fractional parts.

In decimal fractions, a zero is written to the left of the decimal point to indicate clearly that there are no whole numbers in the decimal, just fractional parts, for example, 0.75 (not .75).

DECIMAL FRACTION PLACE VALUE CHART

Whole Number				Fractional Part			
Thousands 1000	Hundreds 100	Tens 10	Units 1	Tenths $\frac{1}{10}$	Hundredths $\frac{1}{100}$	Thousandths $\frac{1}{1000}$	Ten-thousandths $\frac{1}{10,000}$
			0	3	2	5	4

First, look at the fractional parts. Let's add a zero after the last digit to the right of the decimal point.

DECIMAL	COMMON FRACTION	WORDS
0.6	$\frac{6}{10}$	6 tenths
0.60	$\frac{60}{100}$	60 hundredths
0.600	$\frac{600}{1000}$	600 thousandths

Notice here that adding zeroes after the last digit to the right of the decimal point *does not* change the value.

In this example, $0.6 = 0.60 = 0.600$ and $\frac{6}{10} = \frac{60}{100} = \frac{600}{1000}$. Recall from the fraction unit that $\frac{6}{10}$ is in *lower terms* than $\frac{60}{100}$ or $\frac{600}{1000}$. However, $\frac{6}{10}$ is not in *lowest* terms.

Let's put the zero in a different position.

DECIMAL	COMMON FRACTION	WORDS
0.7	$\frac{7}{10}$	7 tenths
0.07	$\frac{7}{100}$	7 hundredths
0.007	$\frac{7}{1000}$	7 thousandths

Adding zeroes between the decimal point and the first number to the right of the decimal point *does* change the value.

To express a decimal fraction in words, read the entire number to the right of the decimal point and then the value of the column last occupied on the right.

A. $0.\overline{9}$ 9 tenths $\frac{9}{10}$

tenths

B. 0.05　　　5 hundredths　　　$\frac{5}{100}$

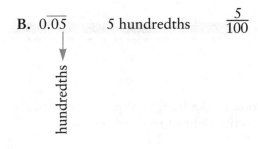

hundredths

C. 0.025　　　25 thousandths　　　$\frac{25}{1000}$

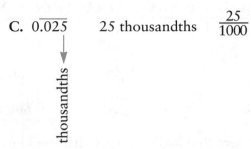

thousandths

　　Decimal fractions may be changed to common fractions by dropping the decimal point to find the numerator, and using the correct denominator.

A. 0.133　　Drop the decimal point and find the numerator of 13. The proper denominator (100) will have as many zeroes as there are decimal places to the right of the decimal point. $0.13 = \frac{13}{100}$

B. 0.2　　　Drop the decimal point and find the numerator of 2. The proper denominator (10) will have as many zeroes as there are decimal places to the right of the decimal point. $0.2 = \frac{2}{10}$

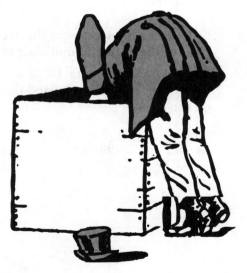

I dropped the decimal point in here someplace but I still can't find the numerator...

C. 0.005   Drop the decimal point and find the numerator of 5. The proper denominator (1000) will have as many zeroes as there are decimal places to the right of the decimal point.
$0.005 = \frac{5}{1000}$

Examine the pairs of equivalent fractions. **The number of zeroes in the common fraction denominator is the same as the number of places to the right of the decimal point in the decimal fraction.**

$0.8 = \frac{8}{10}$ One zero in the denominator.
         One place to the right of the decimal point.

$0.08 = \frac{8}{100}$ Two zeroes in the denominator.
          Two places to the right of the decimal point.

$0.008 = \frac{8}{1000}$ Three zeroes in the denominator.
           Three places to the right of the decimal point.

$0.0008 = \frac{8}{10,000}$ The pattern continues.

To write decimal fractions, think about the common fraction denominator. Again, the number of zeroes in the common fraction denominator is the number of places that must be to the right of the decimal point.

A. Express 2 thousandths as a decimal.
   1. Thousandths has three zeroes in the denominator.
   2. There must be three places to the right of the decimal point.   _ . _ _ _
   3. Put the number 2 in the blank farthest to the right.   0 . _ _ 2
   4. Hold the tenths and hundredths places with zeroes.   0 . 0 0 2

B. Express 4 hundredths as a decimal.
   1. Hundredths has two zeroes in the denominator.   _ . _ _
   2. There must be two places to the right of the decimal point.   0 . _ 4
   3. Put the number 4 in the blank farthest to the right.   0 . 0 4
   4. Hold the tenths place with a zero.

C. Express 6 tenths as a decimal.   _ . _
   1. Tenths has one zero in the denominator.
   2. There must be one place to the right of the decimal point.   0 . 6
   3. Put the number 6 in the tenths column.

D. Write $\frac{16}{1000}$ as a decimal.

    1. There must be three places to the right of the decimal point.   _ . _ _ _

    2. Put the number 16 in the places farthest to the right.   0 . _ 1 6

    3. Hold the tenths place with a zero.   0 . 0 1 6

E. Write $\frac{15}{100}$ as a decimal.

    1. There must be two places to the right of the decimal point.   _ . _ _

    2. Put the number 15 in the blanks.   0 . 1 5

F. This one is *not tricky* if the pattern is followed. Write $\frac{125}{100}$ as a decimal.

    1. There must be two places to the right of the decimal point.   _ . _ _

    2. To put the number 125 in the blanks with only two places to the right of the decimal point, the 1 ends up in the units place.   1 . 2 5

    3. $\frac{125}{100} = 1\frac{25}{100} = 1.25$

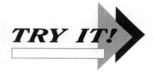

PRACTICE

Fill in the missing elements of the chart.

DECIMAL	WORDS	COMMON FRACTION	LOWEST TERMS OF THE COMMON FRACTION
EXAMPLE 0.75	75 hundredths	$\frac{75}{100}$	$\frac{3}{4}$
1. _____	_____	$\frac{25}{1000}$	_____
2. _____	2 hundredths	_____	_____
3. 0.25	_____	_____	_____
4. _____	_____	$\frac{6}{10}$	_____

Mixed Decimals

Mixed decimals consist of a decimal point and numbers to the right and left of the decimal point (16.2, 8.03, and 5.125). The number to the left of the decimal point represents a whole number. The number to the right of the decimal point represents fractional parts of a whole.

A place value chart for mixed decimals is the same as that used for whole numbers, but it is expanded to the right for the fractional part of a whole. When expressing mixed decimals in words, read the decimal point as "and" to separate the wholes from the fractional part.

DECIMAL FRACTION PLACE VALUE CHART

Whole Number				Fractional Part				
Thousands 1000	Hundreds 100	Tens 10	Units 1	Tenths $\frac{1}{10}$	Hundredths $\frac{1}{100}$	Thousandths $\frac{1}{1000}$	Ten-thousandths $\frac{1}{10,000}$	
		1	6	2				16 and 2 tenths
			8	0	3			8 and 3 hundredths
			5	1	0	5		5 and 105 thousandths

Mixed numbers can be written as decimals. Follow the same pattern used with common fractions. The whole number goes to the left of the decimal point and the fractional part goes to the right. "And" is written as the decimal point.

A. $2\frac{4}{100}$ =   2 . 0 4

B. $17\frac{1}{10}$ =   1 7 . 1

C. $5\frac{12}{1000}$ =   5 . 0 1 2

D. 10 and 6 tenths   =   1 0 . 6

E. 4 and 7 hundredths   =   4 . 0 7

F. 7 and 525 thousandths   =   7 . 5 2 5

From this point on, both decimal fractions and mixed decimals will simply be referred to as decimals. Whole numbers are decimals, too. The decimal system is based on the number 10, as can be seen from the place value chart (0.7, 4., and 4.7).

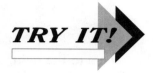

PRACTICE

Fill in the missing elements of the chart.

DECIMAL	WORDS	MIXED NUMBER or COMMON FRACTION
EXAMPLE		
1.05	1 and 5 hundredths	$1\frac{5}{100}$
4.017	4 and 17 thousandths	$4\frac{17}{1000}$
1. _____	_____	$8\frac{9}{100}$
2. _____	2 and 15 thousandths	_____
3. 2.8	_____	_____
4. _____	_____	$4\frac{50}{100}$

ANSWERS

1. 8.09 = 8 and 9 hundredths = $8\frac{9}{100}$
2. 2.015 = 2 and 15 thousandths = $2\frac{15}{1000}$
3. 2.8 = 2 and 8 tenths = $2\frac{8}{10}$
4. 4.50 = 4 and 50 hundredths = $4\frac{50}{100}$

ADDITIONAL PRACTICE

Express each decimal in words. Use "and" for the decimal point in mixed decimals; not in decimal fractions.

5. 0.004 _____

6. 15.125 _____

7. 7.40 _____

8. 0.09 _____

9. 20.02 _____

Express each decimal as a common fraction or mixed number. Then simplify, if possible.

10. 4.5   _____   _____

11. 0.25   _____   _____

12. 16.03   _____   _____

13. 50.04   _____   _____

14. 0.8   _____   _____

Express each of the following as a decimal.

15. $12 \frac{7}{10}$ _____

16. $\frac{12}{100}$ _____

17. $2 \frac{70}{1000}$ _____

18. $145 \frac{3}{100}$ _____

19. $\frac{15}{1000}$ _____

◆◆◆◆◆◆ **FUN FACTS** ◆◆◆◆◆◆

Each year about three thousandths (0.003) of all the surface water on the earth evaporates.

OBJECTIVE

Compare decimals using =, <, OR >.

It is often necessary to know the relative values of two numbers. The procedure for comparing decimal fractions or mixed decimals is similar to the method used for comparing whole numbers.

Comparing Decimals

Begin comparing place value columns from the farthest LEFT. Continue moving to the right in corresponding place value columns until unequal values are found. As soon as unequal values are found in corresponding columns, it is unnecessary to proceed any further to the right. Now, compare 6.95 and 6.9 and find out which one is bigger.

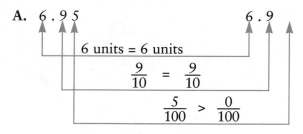

6.95 > 6.9

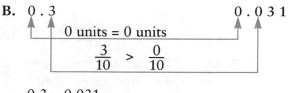

0.3 > 0.031

C. 2.99   3.01

2 < 3

2.99 < 3.01

Also, remember that adding zeroes after the last digit on the right of the decimal point does not change the VALUE of a decimal. When comparing decimals that do not have the same number of decimal places to the right of the decimal point, add zeroes to make the number of decimal places equal. Then compare.

A. Compare 5.06 and 5.063

Add a zero to 5.06 which does not change the value.   5.060

$5.060 < 5.063$ because $5 \frac{60}{1000} < 5 \frac{63}{1000}$.

B. Compare 0.15 and 0.150

Add a zero to 0.15 which does not change the value.   0.150

$0.150 = 0.150$

C. Compare 0.5 to 0.05

Add one zero to 0.5 which does not change the value.   0.50

$0.50 > 0.05$ because $\frac{50}{100} > \frac{5}{100}$.

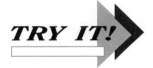

TRY IT!

PRACTICE

Use the symbols =, >, or < to compare the following decimals.

EXAMPLE	$0.31 = 0.3100$

1. 6.419   6.41
2. 0.005   0.011
3. 2.62   3.07
4. 5.6   5.600

ANSWERS
1. $6.419 > 6.41$
2. $0.005 < 0.011$
3. $2.62 < 3.07$
4. $5.6 = 5.600$

ADDITIONAL PRACTICE

Compare each pair of decimals using the symbols =, <, or >.

5. 0.321   0.32   6. 6.415   7.415
7. 3.87   3.789   8. 0.6   0.82
9. 5.3   5.300   10. 7.0   7.01
11. 2.341   2.034   12. 0.009   0.01
13. 0.398   3.98   14. 6.05   6.0500

The volume of four samples was recorded in the laboratory.

Sample W:	0.15 liters
Sample X:	1.05 liters
Sample Y:	1.15 liters
Sample Z:	0.51 liters

1. Which sample is the largest? _____
2. Which sample is the smallest? _____

The lengths of four babies are recorded.

Baby Alan:	45.025 centimeters
Baby Bart:	45.521 centimeters
Baby Connie:	45.125 centimeters
Baby David:	45.052 centimeters

3. Which baby is the longest? _____
4. Which baby is the shortest? _____
5. Two patients receive the same medication. Patient A receives 0.225 gram and Patient B receives 0.125 gram. Which patient receives the smaller dose? _____

PART 3: CONVERTING FRACTIONS TO DECIMALS

OBJECTIVES

1. *Convert a fraction to a decimal.*
2. *Divide decimals by powers of 10 by moving the decimal point to the left.*
3. *Multiply decimals by powers of 10 by moving the decimal point to the right.*

When it is necessary to change a common fraction to a decimal, the fraction bar tells us exactly what to do. The numerator divided by the denominator results in a decimal.

Changing Fractions to Decimals

It is not difficult to express a common fraction as a decimal if the common fraction has a denominator that is a power of 10 (10, 100, 1000, etc.). That, however, is not always the case.

To change any common fraction to its decimal equivalent, divide the numerator by the denominator. Remember, the fraction bar means "divided by."

$$\frac{1}{2} = 1 \div 2 \qquad 2\overline{)\begin{array}{c} .5 \\ 1.0 \\ \underline{1\ 0} \\ 0 \end{array}} \qquad \frac{1}{2} = 0.5$$

$$\frac{3}{5} = 3 \div 5 \qquad 5\overline{)\begin{array}{c} .6 \\ 3.0 \\ \underline{3.0} \\ 0 \end{array}} \qquad \frac{3}{5} = 0.6$$

$$\frac{5}{8} = 5 \div 8 \qquad 8\overline{)\begin{array}{c} .625 \\ 5.000 \\ \underline{4\ 8} \\ 20 \\ \underline{16} \\ 40 \\ \underline{40} \\ 0 \end{array}} \qquad \frac{5}{8} = 0.625$$

Just as $\frac{7}{10}$ is "7 tenths" and is converted to 0.7, the rule above still applies. Divide the numerator by the denominator to change a common fraction to a decimal.

$$\frac{7}{10} = 7 \div 10 \qquad 10\overline{)\begin{array}{c} .7 \\ 7.0 \\ \underline{7\,0} \\ 0 \end{array}} \qquad \frac{7}{10} = 0.7$$

$$\frac{7}{100} = 7 \div 100 \qquad 100\overline{)\begin{array}{c} .07 \\ 7.00 \\ \underline{7\,00} \\ 0 \end{array}} \qquad \frac{7}{100} = 0.07$$

$$\frac{7}{1000} = 7 \div 1000 \qquad 1000\overline{)\begin{array}{c} .007 \\ 7.000 \\ \underline{7\,000} \\ 0 \end{array}} \qquad \frac{7}{1000} = 0.007$$

Notice that something special happened when dividing by a power of 10 (10, 100, 1000, etc.). The number 7 actually has a decimal point to its right (7.), even though decimal points are not normally written next to whole numbers.

A. When 7 is divided by 10, the decimal point moves one place to the left.

$$7. \div 10 = 0.7 \qquad (\,7.\,)$$

B. When 7 is divided by 100, the decimal point moves two places to the left.

$$7 \div 100 = 0.07 \qquad (\,07.\,)$$

C. When 7 is divided by 1000, the decimal point moves three places to the left.

$$7 \div 1000 = 0.007 \qquad (\,007.\,)$$

D. When 24.5 is divided by 100, the decimal point moves two places to the left.

$$24.5 \div 100 = 0.245 \qquad (\,24.5\,)$$

E. When 0.09 is divided by 10, the decimal point moves one place to the left.

$$0.09 \div 10 = 0.009 \qquad (\,0.09\,)$$

To divide any number by a power of 10, move the decimal point to the left the same number of places as there are zeroes in the power of ten.

In a similar manner, it is possible to multiply by powers of 10.

A. 7 x 10 = 70

      7.0 = 70

Move the decimal point one place to the right.

B. 0.09 x 1000 = 90

      0.090 = 90

Move the decimal point three places to the right.

C. 6.259 x 100 = 625.9

      6.259 = 625.9

Move the decimal point two places to the right.

To multiply any number by a power of 10, move the decimal point to the right the same number of places as there are zeroes in the power of ten.

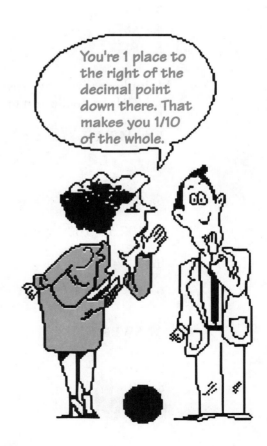

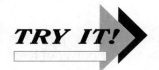

TRY IT!

Change each fraction to a decimal. Remember, numerator divided by denominator.

EXAMPLES	$\frac{6}{4}$ = 1.5
	$2\frac{3}{4}$ = 2.75

1. $\frac{19}{8}$ _____

2. $\frac{3}{4}$ _____

3. $5\frac{1}{8}$ _____

4. $\frac{7}{8}$ _____

5. $\frac{11}{100}$ _____

ANSWERS
1. 2.375
2. 0.75
3. 5.125
4. 0.875
5. 0.11

Multiply or divide by powers of 10 by moving the decimal point. Move to the left to divide and move to the right to multiply.

EXAMPLES	$62.5 \div 10 = 6.25$
	$85 \times 100 = 8500$

6. $0.75 \div 10$ = _____

7. $107.5 \div 100$ = _____

8. 0.07×1000 = _____

9. 1.4×100 = _____

ANSWERS
6. 0.075
7. 1.075
8. 70
9. 140

ADDITIONAL PRACTICE

Convert the following fractions to decimals.

10. $\frac{3}{150}$ = _____   11. $\frac{1}{2}$ = _____

12. $\frac{24}{100}$ = _____   13. $\frac{2}{25}$ = _____

14. $\frac{3}{4}$ = _____   15. $\frac{1}{20}$ = _____

16. $\frac{6}{10}$ = _____   17. $\frac{2}{200}$ = _____

18. $\frac{4}{1000}$ = _____   19. $\frac{3}{8}$ = _____

20. $\frac{3}{5}$ = _____   21. $\frac{7}{8}$ = _____

22. $\frac{1}{5}$ = _____   23. $\frac{9}{100}$ = _____

24. $\frac{1}{8}$ = _____   25. $\frac{4}{5}$ = _____

26. $\frac{1}{10}$ = _____   27. $\frac{5}{8}$ = _____

28. $\frac{25}{1000}$ = _____   29. $\frac{4}{8}$ = _____

Divide the decimals by moving the decimal point.

30. $0.06 \div 100$ = _____

31. $4.34 \div 10$ = _____

32. $12.7 \div 1000$ = _____

33. $0.9 \div 100$ = _____

34. $20.456 \div 10$ = _____

Multiply the decimals by moving the decimal point.

35. 0.95×1000 = _____

36. 4.8×100 = _____

37. 0.741×10 = _____

38. 29.6×10 = _____

39. 0.954×100 = _____

Decimals, not fractions, are always used with metric measurements. Correct the following measurements by stating the fractions in decimal form.

1. $1\frac{3}{4}$ liters   =   _____ liters

2. $2\frac{1}{2}$ grams   =   _____ grams

3. $1\frac{2}{5}$ meters   =   _____ meters

4. $5\frac{7}{8}$ kilograms   =   _____ kilograms

5. $3\frac{1}{8}$ meters   =   _____ meters

◆◆◆◆◆◆ FUN FACTS ◆◆◆◆◆◆◆

The word *decimate* is derived from Latin. It originally referred to a Roman military practice of punishing a troop of men for disobedience by ordering one soldier out of every 10 to be killed.

PART 4: ROUNDING DECIMALS

OBJECTIVES

1. *Round decimals to the nearest tenth.*
2. *Round decimals to the nearest hundredth.*

A rounded number is an approximation for another number. It is often necessary to round if a number has more decimal places than will be required. For most medical calculations, it is only necessary to carry decimals out to the thousandths place and round back to the hundredths place or carry decimals out to hundredths and round back to tenths.

Rounding Decimals

The symbol (~) used with rounded numbers means "is approximately equal to."

6.75 is approximately equal to 6.8   6.75 ~ 6.8

Review the place value chart for decimals.

DECIMAL FRACTION PLACE VALUE CHART

Whole Number				Fractional Part			
Thousands 1000	Hundreds 100	Tens 10	Units 1	Tenths $\frac{1}{10}$	Hundredths $\frac{1}{100}$	Thousandths $\frac{1}{1000}$	Ten-thousandths $\frac{1}{10,000}$

To round a decimal to the nearest *tenth*:

1. Look one place to the right of tenths (that is hundredths).
2. If the hundredths place is 5 or more, increase the tenths by 1, and drop off all digits to the right of tenths.
3. If the hundredths place is 4 or less, leave the tenths alone and drop off all digits to the right of tenths.

A. Round 3.752 to the nearest *tenth*.
    Look one place to the right of tenths.   3.752
    If the hundredths place is 5 or more, increase the tenths by 1, and drop off all digits to the right of tenths.   3.752 ~ 3.8

B. Round 18.62 to the nearest *tenth*.
    Look one place to the right of tenths.   18.62
    If the hundredths place is 4 or less, leave the tenths alone and drop off all digits to the right of tenths.   18.62 ~ 18.6

To round a decimal to the nearest *hundredth*:

1. Look one place to the right of hundredths (that is thousandths).
2. If the thousandths place is 5 or more, increase the hundredths by 1, and drop all digits to the right of hundredths.
3. If the thousandths place is 4 or less, leave the hundredths alone, and drop all the digits to the right of hundredths.

A. Round 0.8725 to the nearest hundredth.
   Look one place to the right of hundredths.   0.8725
      If the thousandths place is 4 or less,
      leave the hundredths alone and drop off
      all digits to the right of hundredths.   0.8725 ~ 0.87

B. Round 4.728 to the nearest hundredth.
   Look one place to the right of hundredths.   4.728
      If the thousandths place is 5 or more, in-
      crease the hundredths by 1, and drop off
      all digits to the right of hundredths.   4.728 ~ 4.73

After a number has been rounded to the nearest tenth, the tenths digit must be the last one showing on the right. After a number has been rounded to the nearest hundredth, the hundredths digit must be the last one showing on the right. Look at these situations.

A. Round 8.996 to the nearest tenth. Look one
   place to the right of tenths.   8.996
      Since the hundredths is five or more, in-
      crease the tenths by 1. Notice what hap-
      pens to the tenths and the whole number.   8.996 ~ 9.0

B. Round 8.996 to the nearest hundredth.
   Look one place to the right of hundredths.   8.996
      Since the thousandths is 5 or more, in-
      crease the hundredths by 1. Notice what
      happens to the hundredths, tenths, and   8.996 ~ 9.00
      whole number.

The skill of rounding can be used in changing fractions to decimals. When dividing the numerator by the denominator, the decimal may terminate (come out even). Or, the decimal may never end no matter how long it is divided. The remainders may repeat and repeat and never come out even.

A. $\dfrac{3}{8} = 3 \div 8$

$$
\begin{array}{r}
.375 \\
8\overline{)3.000} \\
\underline{2\,4} \\
60 \\
\underline{56} \\
40 \\
\underline{40} \\
0
\end{array}
$$

B. $\dfrac{1}{7} = 1 \div 7$

$$
\begin{array}{r}
.14285 \\
7\overline{)1.00000} \\
\underline{7} \\
30 \\
\underline{28} \\
20 \\
\underline{14} \\
60 \\
\underline{56} \\
40 \\
\underline{35} \\
5
\end{array}
$$

It is useful to be able to round a repeating decimal. The division must be carried out to the hundredths to be able to round back to the tenths. Likewise, the division must be carried out to the thousandths to be able to round back to the hundredths.

A. Express $\dfrac{2}{3}$ as a decimal, rounded to the nearest hundredth.

$$
\begin{array}{r}
.666 \\
3\overline{)2.000} \\
\underline{1\,8} \\
20 \\
\underline{18} \\
20 \\
\underline{18} \\
2
\end{array}
$$
$\qquad$ $0.666 \sim 0.67$

B. Express $\dfrac{5}{7}$ as a decimal, rounded to the nearest tenth.

$$
\begin{array}{r}
.71 \\
7\overline{)5.00} \\
\underline{49} \\
10 \\
\underline{7} \\
3
\end{array}
$$
$\qquad$ $0.71 \sim 0.7$

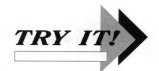

TRY IT!

Round 0.952 to the nearest tenth. _____

Look one place to the right of tenths. It is 5 or more. Increase the tenths by 1, and drop all digits to the right of tenths.	0.952
	0.952 ~ 1.0

Round 0.952 to the nearest hundredth. _____

Look one place to the right of hundredths. It is 4 or less. Leave the hundredths alone and drop all digits to the right of hundredths.	0.952
	0.952 ~ 0.95

PRACTICE

1. Round 0.287 to the nearest tenth. _____

2. Round 6.498 to the nearest hundredth. _____

3. Change $\frac{5}{6}$ to a decimal that is rounded to the nearest tenth. _____

4. Change $\frac{5}{9}$ to a decimal that is rounded to the nearest hundredth. _____

ANSWERS

1. 0.287	~	0.3
2. 6.498	~	6.50
3. $\frac{5}{6}$	~	0.8
4. $\frac{5}{9}$	~	0.56

ADDITIONAL PRACTICE

Round to the nearest tenth.

5. 0.36 _____

6. 4.529 _____

7. 0.97 _____

8. 6.904 _____

9. 11.85 _____

Round to the nearest hundredth.

10. 0.2151 _____

11. 7.991 _____

12. 8.998 _____

13. 15.0062 _____

14. 0.297 _____

Change the fraction to a decimal that is rounded to the nearest hundredth.

15. $\frac{5}{12}$ _____

16. $\frac{2}{11}$ _____

17. $\frac{1}{6}$ _____

18. $\frac{2}{7}$ _____

19. $\frac{8}{7}$ _____

ON THE JOB

The lengths of five babies are recorded. Round the length to the nearest tenth of a centimeter.

1. Baby Anthony: 43.75 centimeters = _____ centimeters
2. Baby Betty: 44.62 centimeters = _____ centimeters
3. Baby Chloe: 47.09 centimeters = _____ centimeters
4. Baby Daniel: 45.125 centimeters = _____ centimeters
5. Baby Elizabeth: 45.99 centimeters = _____ centimeters

The weights of five babies are recorded. Round the weight of each baby to the nearest hundredth.

6. Baby Frank: 3.997 kilograms = _____ kilograms
7. Baby Gloria: 4.002 kilograms = _____ kilograms
8. Baby Henry: 4.255 kilograms = _____ kilograms
9. Baby Ira: 3.906 kilograms = _____ kilograms
10. Baby Jack: 4.593 kilograms = _____ kilograms

PART 5: ADDITION AND SUBTRACTION OF DECIMALS

OBJECTIVES

1. *Add decimal numbers.*
2. *Subtract decimal numbers.*

Whole numbers (which are decimals) are aligned when adding or subtracting so that all hundreds are in one column, tens in another column, and ones in another. (There is a decimal point immediately to the right of a whole number, even though it is not normally used.) Decimal fractions and mixed decimals are also added or subtracted after lining up the decimal points.

Adding Decimal Numbers

To add any decimal numbers, line up the decimal points. To avoid confusion, add zeroes after the last digit to make all of the decimal fractions the same length. This does not change the value of the decimal fraction.

A. 17 + 4 + 125 = _____

$$
\begin{array}{r}
7. \\
4. \\
+\ 125. \\
\hline
136. \\
\end{array}
$$

B. 8.45 + 7.98 = _____

$$
\begin{array}{r}
8.45 \\
+\ 7.98 \\
\hline
16.43 \\
\end{array}
$$

C. 6.94 + 0.5 + 17.102 + 8 = _____

$$
\begin{array}{r}
6.940 \\
0.500 \\
17.102 \\
+\ 8.000 \\
\hline
32.542 \\
\end{array}
$$

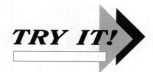

PRACTICE

Line up the decimal points and find the sum.

1. 6.8 + 0.29 + 3   =   _____

2. 0.951 + 6 + 8.24   =   _____

3. 8.9 + 0.03   =   _____

ANSWERS

1. 10.09   2. 15.191   3. 8.93

Subtracting Decimal Numbers

To subtract any decimal numbers, line up the decimal points. To avoid confusion, add zeroes after the last digit to make all of the decimal fractions the same length. This does not change the value of the decimal fraction.

A. 172 – 4 = _____

$$\begin{array}{r} 172. \\ -\ \ \ 4. \\ \hline 168. \end{array}$$

B. 8.4 – 0.7 = _____

$$\begin{array}{r} 8.4 \\ -\ 0.7 \\ \hline 7.7 \end{array}$$

C. 7.8 – 3.92 = _____

$$\begin{array}{r} 7.80 \\ -\ 3.92 \\ \hline 3.88 \end{array}$$

D. 6 – 3.45 = _____

$$\begin{array}{r} 6.00 \\ -\ 3.45 \\ \hline 2.55 \end{array}$$

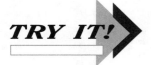

PRACTICE
Line up the decimal points and find the difference.

1. 12 – 3.97   =   _____

2. 8.21 – 4.216   =   _____

3. 16.24 – 5   =   _____

ANSWERS
1. 8.03
2. 3.994
3. 11.24

ADDITIONAL PRACTICE
Find the sum.

4. 0.7 + 0.9 + 0.8   =   _____

5. 7.5 + 16.9 + 25.6   =   _____

6. 0.98 + 4.25 + 6.49   =   _____

7. 6 + 0.4 + 2.3   =   _____

8. $2.96 + 0.8 + 0.45$ = _____

9. $17 + 6.2 + 9.850$ = _____

10. $25.02 + 32$ = _____

11. $0.895 + 0.62 + 5$ = _____

12. $3.9 + 0.12$ = _____

13. $2.85 + 9 + 0.754$ = _____

14. $6 + 8.7 + 72.34$ = _____

15. $47.9 + 307.52$ = _____

Find the difference.

16. $8.2 - 0.79$ = _____

17. $0.5 - 0.479$ = _____

18. $0.479 - 0.3$ = _____

19. $0.74 - 0.58$ = _____

20. $12 - 4.3$ = _____

21. $6 - 3.987$ = _____

22. $4.7 - 0.79$ = _____

23. $25.7 - 19$ = _____

24. $0.342 - 0.178$ = _____

25. $0.95 - 0.826$ = _____

26. $8.3 - 7.9$ = _____

27. $57.04 - 29.38$ = _____

1. A patient receives the following doses of medication: 1.75 milliliters, 2.5 milliliters, and 2 milliliters. What is the total dosage? _____

2. A vial contains 3.5 milliliters of medication. An injection of 2.25 milliliters is withdrawn from the vial into a syringe. How much medication remains in the vial? _____

3. Patient Smith weighed 65.95 kilograms 2 months ago. Her weight then increased by 0.9 kilogram one month, and 1.58 kilograms the next month. What is her current weight? _____

4. Two tablets with a strength of 2.25 milligrams each were administered. What was the total dosage administered? _____

5. Patient Jones weighed 86.59 kilograms. Patient Brown weighed 87.055 kilograms. What is the difference in their weights? _____

6. If three tablets labeled 0.02 milligram each are given, what is the total dosage? _____

7. One tablet is labeled 0.25 milligram and another is labeled 0.5 milligram. What is the total dosage of these two tablets? _____

8. A patient's normal body temperature is 98.6 degrees Fahrenheit. How many degrees above normal is a temperature of 101 degrees? _____

9. A patient is to receive a dosage of 8.5 milligrams. Only 3.75 milligrams has been administered so far. How many more milligrams must be given to this patient? _____

10. A patient is to receive a dosage of 2.5 milligrams and has been given 1.75 milligrams. What additional amount of medication must be administered? _____

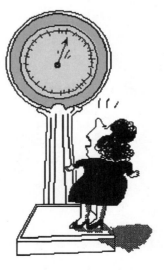

65.95 kilograms plus 0.9 kilogram plus 1.58 kilograms means rabbit food for the next few months!

OBJECTIVE

Multiply decimals.

The procedure for multiplying decimals is the same as for whole numbers. However, before finding the answer (the answer is called the *product* in multiplication), certain rules must be followed.

Multiplying Decimals

Observe the names given to the parts of a multiplication problem.

Factor	x	Factor	=	Product
0.2	x	0.4	=	0.08

To multiply decimals, multiply the factors as if they were whole numbers. Total the number of decimal places to the right of the decimal point in *both* factors. Insert the decimal point in the answer so that the same number of decimal places are to the right of the decimal point as in *both* factors together.

A.
$$\begin{array}{r} 6.51 \\ \times \quad .2 \\ \hline 1.302 \end{array}$$

(2 decimal places)
(1 decimal place)
(3 decimal places)

B.
$$\begin{array}{r} 30.7 \\ \times \ 1.6 \\ \hline 1842 \\ 307 \ \\ \hline 49.12 \end{array}$$

(1 decimal place)
(1 decimal place)

(2 decimal places)

C.
$$\begin{array}{r} 7.9 \\ \times \ 12. \\ \hline 158 \\ 79 \ \\ \hline 94.8 \end{array}$$

(1 decimal place)
(0 decimal places)

(1 decimal place)

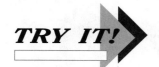

TRY IT!

PRACTICE

Multiply to find the product. Round the answer to the nearest hundredth if necessary.

> **EXAMPLE**   6.95 x 11 = 76.45

1. 0.03 x 0.2   =   _____

2. 14 x 52.1   =   _____

3. 0.81 x 7.9   =   _____

4. 0.05 x 0.7   =   _____

ANSWERS
1. 0.006 ~ 0.01
2. 729.4
3. 6.399 ~ 6.40
4. 0.035 ~ 0.04

ADDITIONAL PRACTICE

Multiply to find the product. Round the answers to the nearest hundredth, if necessary.

5. 0.4 x 9   =   _____

6. 0.05 x 2   =   _____

7. 0.75 x 0.08   =   _____

8. 0.152 x 0.7   =   _____

9. 29 x 0.06   =   _____

10. 15 x 0.007   =   _____

11. 0.53 x 0.2   =   _____

12. 8.45 x 0.75   =   _____

13. 0.256 x 29   =   _____

14. 0.008 x 5   =   _____

15. 0.27 x 0.84   =   _____

16. 0.062 x 0.51   =   _____

Multiply by the power of ten by moving the decimal point.

17. 6.98 x 10   =   _____

18. 52.3 x 100   =   _____

19. 0.08 x 1000   =   _____

20. 4.1 x 100   =   _____

21. 78 x 10   =   _____

ON THE JOB

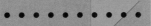

1. A patient is given 0.09 kilogram of meat for each meal. How many kilograms of meat are served in nine meals? _____

2. A container holds 10.75 liters of ethyl alcohol. How much alcohol is in six of these containers? _____

3. There are $3\frac{1}{2}$ (3.5) tablets with a strength of 1.75 milligrams each. How many milligrams are in $3\frac{1}{2}$ tablets? _____

4. The tablets for Patient Campbell are each labeled 0.1 milligram. If this patient is given $2\frac{1}{2}$ tablets, what is the total dosage? _____

5. A single tablet is 12.5 milligrams. If $3\frac{1}{2}$ tablets are administered during one day, what is the total dosage? _____

PART 7: DIVISION OF DECIMALS

OBJECTIVE

Divide decimals.

The procedure for division of decimals is the same as for division of whole numbers. However, certain rules must be followed before dividing so that the quotient is expressed correctly. Division of decimals is different than lining up the decimal points for addition and subtraction or counting decimal places for multiplication.

Division of Decimals

Observe the names given to the parts of a division problem.

$$\frac{\text{dividend}}{\text{divisor}} = \text{quotient} \qquad \frac{3}{2} = 1.5$$

$$\text{dividend} \div \text{divisor} = \text{quotient}$$
$$3 \div 2 = 1.5$$

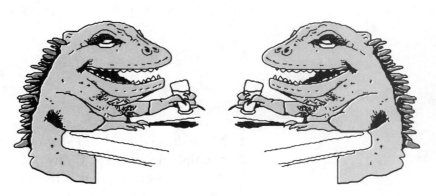

Remember: *Quotient* is another name for *Answer*.
They're one and the same.

If the divisor is a whole number, place the decimal point in the quotient directly above the decimal point in the dividend. Then divide. Look at the following examples.

A. $1.26 \div 6 = \dfrac{1.26}{6}$

$$
\begin{array}{r}
.21 \\
6\overline{)1.26} \\
\underline{1\,2} \\
6 \\
\underline{6} \\
0
\end{array}
$$

$$\text{B. } 51.2 \div 8 = \frac{51.2}{8} \qquad \begin{array}{r} 6.4 \\ 8\overline{)51.2} \\ \underline{48} \\ 3\ 2 \\ \underline{3\ 2} \\ 0 \end{array}$$

$$\text{C. } 7 \div 8 = \frac{7}{8} \qquad \begin{array}{r} .875 \\ 8\overline{)7.000} \\ \underline{6\ 4} \\ 60 \\ \underline{56} \\ 40 \\ \underline{40} \\ 0 \end{array}$$

If the divisor is not a whole number, move the decimal point the same number of places to the right in the divisor and the dividend so that the divisor becomes a whole number. Place the decimal point in the quotient directly above the new decimal point in the dividend. Then divide.

$$\text{A. } 7 \div 1.75 = \frac{7}{1.75} \qquad \begin{array}{r} 4. \\ 1.75\overline{)7.00} \\ \underline{7\ 00} \\ 0 \end{array}$$

1. Make the divisor (1.75) a whole number by multiplying times 100.
2. Multiply the dividend (7) by the same number, 100.
3. Place the decimal point in the quotient (your answer).
4. Divide.

Moving the decimal point the same number of places to the right in the divisor and the dividend is the same as multiplying them each by the same power of ten. Multiplying the numerator (dividend) and denominator (divisor) by the same number does not change the value of the fraction.

$$\frac{7}{1.75} \times \frac{100}{100} = \frac{700}{175} = 4$$

B. $14.48 \div 0.4$ $=$ $\dfrac{14.48}{0.4}$

$$0.4\,\overline{)14.48} \quad \begin{array}{r} 36.2 \\ \hline \end{array}$$

```
        36.2
0.4)14.48
    12
    ‾‾
     2 4
     2 4
     ‾‾‾
       08
       08
       ‾‾
        0
```

1. Make the divisor (0.4) a whole number by multiplying by 10.
2. Multiply the dividend (14.48) by the same number, 10.
3. Place the decimal point in the quotient.
4. Divide.

C. $0.006 \div 1.2$ $=$ $\dfrac{0.006}{1.2}$

```
         .005
1.2)0.0060
```

D. $31.5 \div 0.015$ $=$ $\dfrac{31.5}{0.015}$

```
             2 100.
0.015)31.500
      30
      ‾‾
       1 5
       1 5
       ‾‾‾
         0
```

E. $0.448 \div 3.2$ $=$ $\dfrac{0.448}{3.2}$

```
         0.14
3.2)0.4 48
    3 2
    ‾‾
    1 28
    1 28
    ‾‾‾‾
       0
```

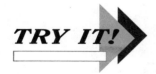 **TRY IT!**

PRACTICE

Divide to find the quotient. Round the answer to the nearest hundredth, if necessary. (To be able to round to the nearest hundredth, the quotient must be carried out to the thousandths place first.)

EXAMPLE	$16 \div 0.02$	$=$	800

1. $0.04 \div 0.3$ $=$ _____

2. $0.175 \div 25$ $=$ _____

3. $0.375 \div 1.25$ $=$ _____

4. $15 \div 2.6$ $=$ _____

ADDITIONAL PRACTICE

Divide to find the quotient. Round the answers to the nearest hundredth, if necessary.

5. $8.89 \div 7$ = _____

6. $12 \div 1.4$ = _____

7. $0.736 \div 8$ = _____

8. $15 \div 6$ = _____

9. $4.12 \div 3.09$ = _____

10. $82.5 \div 25.4$ = _____

11. $49 \div 2.8$ = _____

12. $0.06 \div 0.09$ = _____

13. $2.7 \div 0.009$ = _____

14. $41.1 \div 2.1$ = _____

15. $7.9 \div 0.025$ = _____

16. $0.09 \div 12$ = _____

Divide by the power of 10 by moving the decimal point.

17. $5.9 \div 10$ = _____

18. $6.89 \div 100$ = _____

19. $49.6 \div 1000$ = _____

20. $2 \div 100$ = _____

21. $75 \div 1000$ = _____

1. A container holds 16.25 milliliters of medication. How many 1.25 milliliter doses can be administered from this container? _____

2. Four babies were born during a two-week period. The weights of the babies are as follows:

   Baby Keith: 3.551 kilograms
   Baby Matt: 3.497 kilograms
   Baby Laurie: 4.212 kilograms
   Baby Nancy: 4.625 kilograms

   Find the average weight of the four babies, rounded to the nearest hundredth. _____

   (Average = Total weight of the babies ÷ Number of babies)

3. The total prescribed dosage of a medication is 4.5 grams. How many 1.5 gram tablets need to be administered? _____

4. A medication has 2.25 grams in every two tablets. How many grams are in one tablet? _____

5. How many 0.5 gram doses can be obtained from a 4 gram vial of medication? _____

♦♦♦♦♦♦ **FUN FACTS** ♦♦♦♦♦♦

A slice of skin with a thickness of 0.008 inch is used for a typical skin graft.

EXERCISES

Convert to decimals.

1. $3\frac{2}{5}$ = _____

2. $\frac{3}{4}$ = _____

3. $7\frac{1}{2}$ = _____

4. $\frac{8}{10}$ = _____

5. $\frac{1}{4}$ = _____

6. $\frac{19}{100}$ = _____

7. $4\frac{5}{8}$ = _____

8. $2\frac{14}{1000}$ = _____

9. $\frac{1}{20}$ = _____

10. $7\frac{1}{100}$ = _____

11. $8\frac{1}{10}$ = _____

12. $\frac{3}{5}$ = _____

13. $\frac{9}{12}$ = _____

14. $5\frac{10}{20}$ = _____

15. $\frac{10}{10}$ = _____

16. $\frac{3}{6}$ = _____

Multiply or divide each decimal by the power of ten by moving the decimal point.

17. 7.95×10 = _____

18. $0.04 \div 10$ = _____

19. $62.9 \div 100$ = _____

20. 1.8×1000 = _____

21. $9.8 \div 1000$ = _____

22. $0.8 \div 100$ = _____

23. 0.051×100 = _____

24. 8.2×10 = _____

25. 14.125×100 = _____

26. 49×1000 = _____

Compare the decimals using =, >, or <.

27. 3.87   8.37
28. 0.8   0.785
29. 0.398   0.389
30. 5.6   5.600
31. 0.009   0.02

32. 1.50   1.05
33. 2.7   2.648
34. 0.05   0.050
35. 2.98   0.298
36. 4.089   4.8

UNIT 2 REVIEW

Round each decimal to the nearest tenth.

37. 6.954 = _____	**40.** 0.05 = _____	**43.** 14.947 = _____
38. 0.82 = _____	**41.** 1.91 = _____	**44.** 0.23 = _____
39. 4.399 = _____	**42.** 0.990 = _____	**45.** 100.75 = _____

Round each decimal to the nearest hundredth.

46. 14.046 = _____	**51.** 5.998 = _____
47. 0.0128 = _____	**52.** 0.452 = _____
48. 5.005 = _____	**53.** 0.594 = _____
49. 0.986 = _____	**54.** 8.215 = _____
50. 3.992 = _____	**55.** 12.010 = _____

Add the decimals to find the sum.

56. $0.9 + 4.50 + 12$ = _____	**59.** $7.8 + 9 + 0.62$ = _____
57. $1.4 + 0.8 + 0.755$ = _____	**60.** $150 + 17.5 + 0.99$ = _____
58. $1.8 + 0.95$ = _____	**61.** $17 + 95 + 5.75$ = _____

Subtract the decimals to find the difference.

62. $7.2 - 0.88$ = _____	**65.** $15.75 - 8$ = _____
63. $4.12 - 3.984$ = _____	**66.** $16 - 4.75$ = _____
64. $12 - 6.3$ = _____	**67.** $4.18 - 0.543$ = _____

Multiply the decimals to find the product. Round the product to the nearest hundredth (2 decimal places) if necessary.

68. 14×0.75 = _____	**71.** 9.8×1.5 = _____
69. 1.25×8 = _____	**72.** 8.62×0.28 = _____
70. 0.24×0.65 = _____	**73.** 0.007×16 = _____

Divide the decimals to find the quotient. Round the quotient to the nearest hundredth if necessary.

74. $29.64 \div 3.9$ =   _____

75. $0.245 \div 0.07$ =   _____

76. $73.0184 \div 1.003$ =   _____

77. $2.117 \div 7.3$ =   _____

78. $0.4 \div 0.025$ =   _____

79. $8 \div 3$ =   _____

Solve using the appropriate operation.

80. 0.05×0.9 =   _____

81. $1.75 \div 10$ =   _____

82. $4.7 + 8 + 9.75 + 2.1$ =   _____

83. $16 - 2.641$ =   _____

84. 0.3×1000 =   _____

85. 0.625×10 =   _____

86. $45.9 \div 6.8$ =   _____

87. $4.2 - 3.95$ =   _____

88. $7.9 + 4.55 + 0.029 + 5$ =   _____

89. $76 \div 1000$ =   _____

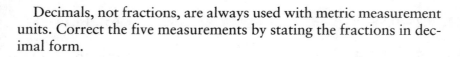

ON THE JOB

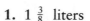

Decimals, not fractions, are always used with metric measurement units. Correct the five measurements by stating the fractions in decimal form.

1. $1 \frac{3}{8}$ liters   =   _____ liters

2. $2 \frac{3}{4}$ meters   =   _____ meters

3. $5 \frac{1}{2}$ grams   =   _____ grams

4. $58 \frac{1}{4}$ kilograms   =   _____ kilograms

5. $75 \frac{4}{5}$ centimeters   =   _____ centimeters

The volume, weight, and length of various samples were recorded in the laboratory. Compare the pairs of measurements using =, <, or >.

6. 2.5 centimeters   2.05 centimeters
7. 79.45 kilograms   79.54 kilograms
8. 71.5 centimeters   71.50 centimeters
9. 8.5 grams   8.49 grams
10. 0.25 milligrams   0.5 milligrams

The lengths of five babies were recorded. Round the length measurements to the nearest tenth.

11. Baby Oscar: 48.75 centimeters   = _____ centimeters
12. Baby Patty: 46.19 centimeters   = _____ centimeters
13. Baby Quentin: 47.04 centimeters   = _____ centimeters
14. Baby Roland: 45.30 centimeters   = _____ centimeters
15. Baby Sue: 44.98 centimeters   = _____ centimeters

The weights of five patients were recorded. Round the weights to the nearest hundredth.

16. Patient Tom: 56.828 kilograms   _____
17. Patient Vicki: 90.909 kilograms   _____
18. Patient Wayne: 84.090 kilograms   _____
19. Patient Adele: 66.363 kilograms   _____
20. Patient Barbara: 72.727 kilograms   _____

21. A patient receives the following doses of medication: 4.5 milliliters, 2.55 milliliters, and 3 milliliters. What is the total dosage? _____

22. The patient is to receive a dosage of 7 milligrams. Only 2.75 milligrams have been administered so far. How many more milligrams must be given to the patient? _____

23. A single tablet is 10.5 milligrams. If $2\frac{1}{2}$ (2.5) tablets are administered, what is the total dosage?

     _____

24. Three tablets, each with a strength of 2.25 milligrams, were given to the patient. What is the total dosage? _____

25. One tablet is labeled 0.5 milligram and another is labeled 1.5 milligrams. What is the total dosage of these two tablets?

     _____

26. Each tablet has a strength of 0.04 milligram. How many milligrams of medication are in $4\frac{1}{4}$ (4.25) tablets? _____

27. A container holds 18.75 milliliters of medication. How many 1.25 milliliter doses can be administered from this container? _____

28. A medicine bottle contains eight doses. How many bottles are necessary for 45 doses? _____

29. If a patient's normal body temperature is 98.6 degrees Fahrenheit, how many degrees above normal is a temperature of 100 degrees? _____

30. Ten patients are each to receive a 2.5 milliliter dose of the same medication. How many milliliters will be needed in all? _____

31. Patient Yousef weighed 86.45 kilograms two months ago. His weight then decreased by 2 kilograms one month and by 1.5 kilograms the next. What does this patient weigh now? _____

32. How many 2.5 milliliter doses can be obtained from a 15 milliliter source? _____

33. A total of 270.9 grams of meat is to be served in three meals. How many grams of meat should be served in each meal? _____

34. A patient drank the following amounts of liquid in four consecutive days: 1.25 liters, 1.6 liters, 1.8 liters, and 1.75 liters. What is the total amount of liquid consumed? _____

35. If a patient's normal body temperature is 98.6 degrees Fahrenheit, how many degrees below normal is a temperature of 96.8 degrees? _____

36. Container A can hold 12.5 liters of liquid. Container B is 0.75 the size of Container A. Container C is 0.5 the size of Container A.

    How much liquid can be stored in Container B? _____

    How much liquid can be stored in Container C? _____

37. A medicine bottle contains 10 doses. How many bottles would be necessary for 38 doses? _____

38. Patient Conors weighed 54 kilograms when admitted to the hospital. In the two weeks since, gains of 0.92 kilogram and 0.5 kilogram have been recorded. What does this patient weigh now? _____

39. A patient's temperature is 2.8 degrees above normal (98.6 degrees Fahrenheit). What is the reading on the thermometer? _____

40. The following doses of a certain medication were given to a patient on Tuesday: 0.5 ounce, 1.5 ounces, and 1.75 ounces. What was the total dosage? _____

UNIT

3 Metric System of Measurement

PART 1: INTRODUCTION TO THE METRIC SYSTEM

OBJECTIVES

1. *Identify the meter as the basic unit of length.*
2. *Identify the liter as the basic unit of volume.*
3. *Identify the gram as the basic unit of weight.*

Simply stated, the metric system is a decimal system based on tens. It is used to measure length, volume, and weight. The basic unit of length is the meter. The basic unit of volume is the liter. The basic unit of weight is the gram.

History

The need to measure size and distance became apparent in even the earliest civilizations. The English measurement system was developed using such units as the yard (length), the gallon (volume), and the pound (weight) to describe the various measures. Although the English system attempted to standardize, there is no logical connection between the basic measurement units. Thus, 36 inches equal a yard, 4 quarts equal a gallon, 16 ounces equal a pound, and so on. There is no order to this system—only a collection of awkwardly related measures.

About 1670 a Frenchman developed a system of measurement organized according to the decimal system of numeration. The system was not officially adopted by France until the late 1790's. It has since been adopted in every other country except the United States. Our country is moving slowly toward the adoption of metrics as its measurement system, but in actual practice the system is used in many types of operations. *In the prescription and administration of drugs, a working knowledge of metrics is imperative.*

Basic Units of Length, Volume, and Weight

The basic unit of length, the meter, is standardized throughout the world. (For reference, it is slightly longer than a yard.) There are other units of length in the metric system, some of which are larger than a meter (kilometer, hectometer, and dekameter) and some of which are smaller than a meter (decimeter, centimeter, and millimeter). *Notice that the word meter appears in all units of length.*

The basic unit of volume, the liter, is defined as the amount of liquid which is contained in a cube which is 10 centimeters long, 10 centimeters wide, and 10 centimeters high. Since VOLUME = LENGTH x WIDTH x HEIGHT, the volume of the cube is stated as 1000 cubic centimeters (1000 cc). Notice that the volume is expressed as 1000 cc (cubic centimeters) or 1 liter. (For reference, the liter is slightly more than a quart.)

There are units of volume that are larger than a liter (kiloliter, hectoliter, and dekaliter) and units that are smaller than a liter (deciliter, centiliter, and milliliter). Remember that volume also can be expressed in cubic measurement (1 milliliter = 1 cubic centimeter or 1 mL = 1 cc). **Whenever the word *liter* appears, it is a measurement of volume.**

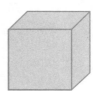

1 mL = 1 cc

The basic unit of weight is the gram. It is a small unit, approximately the weight of two paper clips. There are units of weight that are larger than a gram (kilogram, hectogram, and dekagram) and units that are smaller than a gram (decigram, centigram, and milligram). (The kilogram is about 2.2 pounds.) **Whenever the word *gram* appears, it is a unit of weight.**

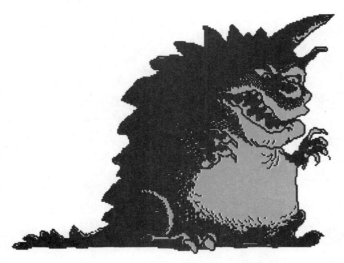

The basic unit of length is the *meter*. The basic unit of volume is the *liter*. The basic unit of weight is the *gram*. Got it? Good.

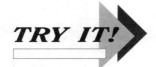

TRY IT!

PRACTICE

1. The metric system of measurement was developed in the country of
   _____. It is a decimal system based on the number _____.

2. The basic unit of length is _____ and the basic unit of weight is a
   _____.

3. The basic unit of volume is a _____ which is equal to 1000 cc (cubic
   centimeters); 1 milliliter equals _____ cc (cubic centimeter).

ANSWERS

1. France, ten
2. meter, gram
3. liter; 1 mL = 1 cc

◆◆◆◆◆◆ **FUN FACTS** ◆◆◆◆◆◆

A gram of venom from the King Cobra is so deadly that it could kill 150 people.

PART 2: METRIC SYMBOLS AND NOTATION

OBJECTIVES

1. *State the six prefixes (and their meanings) that are used with meter, liter, and gram.*
2. *Interpret correct metric notation.*
3. *Write measurements of length, volume, and weight in correct metric notation.*

Specific symbols and guidelines for notation have been adopted to express metric measurements. To prevent confusion, standard metric notation should always be used.

Metric Symbols

In actual use, metric units are shortened to symbols when used with number quantities (6 m , 12.5 L , and 0.5 g). There are no periods, for these are symbols and not abbreviations.

	BASIC UNIT	SYMBOL	
For length	meter	m	
For volume	liter	L	(Liter is symbolized with a capital L to avoid confusion with the number 1.)
For weight	gram	g	

Basically, six main prefixes are used with meter, liter, and gram. Each of the prefixes is symbolized by a single lowercase letter, except deka-. The da is used to avoid confusion with the d which represents deci-.

	PREFIX	SYMBOL
To mean 1000 units	kilo-	k
To mean 100 units	hecto-	h
To mean 10 units	deka-	da
To mean 1 unit		m or L or g (meter, liter, gram)
To mean 0.1 unit	deci-	d
To mean 0.01 unit	centi-	c
To mean 0.001 unit	milli-	m

The symbol of the prefix and the symbol of the basic unit are combined to represent all of the various units of measure. Additionally, the symbol for cubic centimeter (cc) will be used for volume measurements (1 mL = 1 cc). The units with the asterisk (*) are the most commonly used metric units and will be the focus of this text. The others are presented to show the decimal order of the system.

LENGTH	VOLUME	WEIGHT
*kilometer km	kiloliter kL	*kilogram kg
hectometer hm	hectoliter hL	hectogram hg
dekameter dam	dekaliter daL	dekagram dag
*meter m	*liter L	*gram g
decimeter dm	deciliter dL	decigram dg
*centimeter cm	centiliter cL	centigram cg
*millimeter mm	*milliliter mL	*milligram mg

Metric Notation

In the metric system, the numbers are expressed in decimals, not common fractions. A space is left between the number and the symbol. Fractional parts of a unit are written with a zero in the units place to show clearly and unmistakably that there are no wholes.

0.5 mL

1 mL

1.5 mL

Unnecessary zeroes, on the other hand, are eliminated.

1.8 g not 1.80 g

0.75 m not 0.750 m

Digits are separated in groups of three, counting from the decimal point left and the decimal point right. Commas are not used in the metric system.

85 423.167 4 not 85,423.1674

7 125.75 not 7,125.75

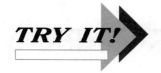

PRACTICE

Write the appropriate symbol.

1. kilogram __K__ centimeter __cm__ millimeter __mm__

2. meter __m__ gram __g__ kilometer __km__

3. liter __L__ milliliter __mL__ milligram __mg__

Express the following in correct metric notation with symbols.

4. 60 hundredths milliliter __.06 mL__

5. 4 grams __4 g__

6. 8210 and $\frac{75}{100}$ meters __8210.75 m__

7. $\frac{600}{1000}$ liter __.06 L__

ANSWERS

1. kg, cm, mm
2. m, g, km
3. L, mL, mg
4. 0.6 mL
5. 4 g
6. 8 210.75 m
7. 0.6 L

ADDITIONAL PRACTICE

Write the correct metric notation, using decimals and symbols.

8. $\frac{75}{100}$ kilogram __.75 kg__

9. 8425 and $\frac{6}{10}$ liters __8425.6 L__

10. $\frac{5}{10}$ hectogram __.5 hg__

11. 6 and $\frac{50}{100}$ centimeters __6.05 cm__

12. $\frac{750}{1000}$ kilometer __.750 km__

13. $1\frac{1}{2}$ milliliters __1.50 mL__

14. 5 dekameters __5 dam__

15. $3\frac{3}{4}$ millimeters __3.75 mm__

16. 27,425 grams _____

17. 3 milliliters __.3 mm__

18. $\frac{6}{10}$ decimeter __.6 dm__

19. 4 and $\frac{12}{1000}$ meters __4.012 m__

20. $7\frac{1}{4}$ hectogram __7.25 hg__

21. 8 and $\frac{7}{100}$ milligrams __8.07 mg__

22. 10 milliliters __.1 mm__

OBJECTIVES

1. *Identify metric units of length that are larger and smaller than the meter.*
2. *List the most commonly used length equivalents within the metric system.*
3. *Convert from one length unit to another within the metric system.*

Seven different metric units of length are presented in this section. The focus of the conversion process in this part, however, is on the most commonly used metric length equivalents.

Metric Length Measurement

A meter (m) is the basic unit of length in the metric system. (Remember that a meter is slightly longer than a yard.)

To express measurement units that are *larger* than a meter, three prefixes are added to the word "meter."

PREFIX	MEANING	SYMBOL
kilo-	1000	k
hecto-	100	h
deka-	10	da

A kilometer (km) is 1000 meters.

A hectometer (hm) is 100 meters.

A dekameter (dam) is 10 meters.

Each unit is 10 times the next smaller unit.

To express measurement units that are *smaller* than a meter, three other prefixes are used.

PREFIX	MEANING	SYMBOL
deci-	0.1 (1/10)	d
centi-	0.01 (1/100)	c
milli-	0.001 (1/1000)	m

A decimeter (dm) is 0.1 meter.   10 decimeters = 1 meter.

A centimeter (cm) is 0.01 meter.   100 centimeters = 1 meter.

A millimeter (mm) is 0.001 meter.   1000 millimeters = 1 meter.

```
  1    2    3    4    5    6    7    8    9   10
|ılıılıılıılıılıılıılıılıılıılıılıılıılıılıılıılıılıılıılıı|
```

Each of the smallest subdivisions shown is a millimeter (mm). Remember that 10 millimeters form a centimeter (cm), 10 centimeters form a decimeter (dm), and 10 decimeters form a meter (m). Each unit is 10 times the next smaller unit.

A meter stick, used to measure the basic unit of length in the metric system, shows millimeter, centimeter, and decimeter subdivisions.

$$1 \text{ m} = 1000 \text{ mm} \qquad 1 \text{ m} = 100 \text{ cm} \qquad 1 \text{ m} = 10 \text{ dm}$$

Six prefixes and the basic unit, the meter, provide seven units of metric length.

Units larger than 1 meter

kilometer	km	=	1000 m
hectometer	hm	=	100 m
dekameter	dam	=	10 m

Unit equal to a meter

meter	m	=	1 m

Units smaller than 1 meter

decimeter	dm	=	0.1 m
centimeter	cm	=	0.01 m
millimeter	mm	=	0.001 m

Metric Length Conversion

After learning the units of length, the next step is to learn how to convert or change from one unit to another within the metric system.

Think back to the English system.

1 foot = 12 inches	The conversion factor from feet to inches is 12.
3 feet = 1 yard	The conversion factor from feet to yards is 3.
1 mile = 1760 yards	The conversion factor from yards to miles is 1760.

Now examine the following table of most commonly used metric length equivalents. This information should be memorized. Notice that the conversion factor in the metric system is always a power of 10, that is, 10 or 100 or 1000, etc.

METRIC LENGTH EQUIVALENTS	
The conversion factor between meter and kilometer is 1000.	1 km = 1000 m
The conversion factor between meter and millimeter is 1000.	1 m = 1000 mm
The conversion factor between meter and centimeter is 100.	1 m = 100 cm
The conversion factor between centimeter and millimeter is 10.	1 cm = 10 mm

There are only two steps in the conversion process:

1. Remember the equivalents. This information provides the conversion factor.

2. Multiply by the conversion factor to convert to smaller units.
   OR
   Divide by the conversion factor to find larger units.

A. _____ m = 2.85 km

   Step 1: Equivalent?

   Remember the meter–kilometer equivalent. 1 km = 1000 m. The conversion factor = 1000.

   Step 2: Multiply or Divide?

   The conversion is to a smaller unit. (Meters are smaller than kilometers.) It will take MORE of the smaller units to make an equivalent amount of the larger units. Multiply by 1000, the conversion factor. Move the decimal point three places to the right to multiply by 1000.

   2 850 m = 2.85 km

B. 25 mm = _____ cm

   Step 1: Equivalent?

   Remember the millimeter–centimeter equivalent. 10 mm = 1 cm. The conversion factor is 10.

   Step 2: Multiply or Divide?

   The conversion is to a larger unit. (A centimeter is larger than a millimeter.) It will take FEWER of the larger units to make an equivalent amount of the smaller units. Divide by 10, the conversion factor. Move the decimal point one place to the left to divide by 10.

   25 mm = 2.5 cm

C. _____ m = 57 mm

   Step 1: Equivalent?

   1 m = 1000 mm   Conversion factor = 1000

   Step 2: Multiply or Divide?

   Divide to convert to a larger unit. Move the decimal point 3 places to the left to divide by 1000.

   0.057 m = 57 mm

D. 0.04 m = _____ cm

   Step 1: Equivalent?

   1 m = 100 cm   Conversion factor = 100

   Step 2: Multiply or Divide ?

   Multiply to convert to a smaller unit. Move the decimal point 2 places to the right to multiply by 100.

   0.04 m = 4 cm

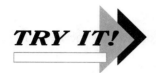

PRACTICE

Convert the following metric length units. Multiply by the conversion factor to change to smaller units. Divide by the conversion factor to change to larger units.

> **EXAMPLES**
>
> 75.1 m = <u>100</u> cm   (7 510 cm)
> (1 m = 100 cm. Multiply by 100 to find smaller units.)
>
> 850 mm = $\dfrac{1}{1000}$ m   (0.85 m)
> (1 m = 1000 mm. Divide by 1000 to find larger units.)

1. 6.9 m   ✗ <u>1000</u> mm

2. 25 mm = _____ ᵐᵐcm
   6.01

3. ____ . ____ km = $\dfrac{765.1\text{ m}}{1000}$

4. 14.7 cm = _____ m
   $\overline{0.01}$

5. _____ cm = $\dfrac{75\text{ mm}}{0.01}$

ANSWERS

1. 6 900 mm
2. 2.5 cm
3. 0.765 1 km
4. 0.147 m
5. 7.5 cm

Going from larger to smaller you multiply

going from smaller to larger you divide

ADDITIONAL PRACTICE

6. Name three units of metric length that are longer than a meter.
   _____ _____ _____

7. Name three units of metric length that are shorter than a meter.
   _____ _____ _____

8. Fill in the blanks to make an equivalent statement.

   _____ cm = 1 mm   _____ cm = 1 m

   _____ m = 1 km   _____ mm = 1 m

   _____ dm = 1 m

Express each measure as an equivalent in a larger or smaller metric unit.

9. 0.45 cm = _____ mm   **10.** 8.5 km = _____ m

11. 95 mm = _____ cm   **12.** 1.5 cm = _____ mm

13. 535 cm = _____ m   **14.** 1495 m = _____ km

15. 78 mm = _____ m   **16.** 45.5 cm = _____ m

17. 89.5 mm = _____ cm   **18.** 6.8 m = _____ cm

19. 78 cm = _____ mm   **20.** 0.29 dm = _____ m

21. 0.42 cm = _____ mm   **22.** 125 mm = _____ m

23. 0.25 km = _____ m   **24.** 15.25 m = _____ dm

25. 4500 m = _____ km

ON THE JOB

The heights of four patients were recorded. Express the measurement in the indicated unit. Round to the nearest hundredth, if necessary.

1. Patient Andrews: 142.5 cm _____ m

2. Patient Bower: 155 cm _____ m

3. Patient Cones: 1.025 m _____ cm

4. Patient Ditmar: 1.75 m _____ cm

5. The range in length of newborn babies is 45–55 centimeters. Express this range in millimeters.

_____ mm – _____ mm

6. During a physical assessment, a mole on a patient's back was noted and measured.

Mole: 21 mm = _____ cm

7. A child was admitted to the emergency room with a cut which was noted in the records.

Cut: 95 mm = _____ cm

PART 4: VOLUME MEASUREMENT AND CONVERSION

OBJECTIVES

1. *Identify metric units of volume that are larger and smaller than the liter.*
2. *Explain how volume can also be expressed in cubic units.*
3. *List the most commonly used volume equivalents within the metric system.*
4. *Convert from one volume unit to another within the system.*

An overview of eight metric volume units is presented in this part. In health care, conversions are made between milliliters and cubic centimeters, milliliters and liters, and liters and cubic centimeters.

Metric Volume

A liter is the basic unit of volume or capacity in the metric system. Remember that a liter is slightly more than a quart. A liter is the amount of liquid that will fill a cube that is 10 cm long, 10 cm wide, and 10 cm high. **This cube that has a volume of 1000 cc holds 1 liter.**

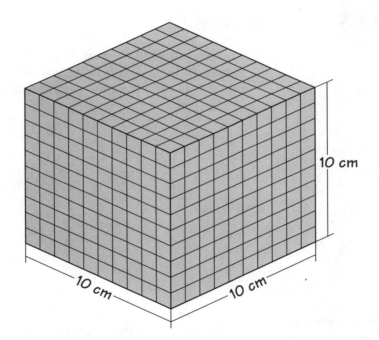

10 cm

10 cm

10 cm

1000 cc = 1 L = 1000 mL
    1 cubic centimeter is 1 cc
    1 cc holds 1 mL of liquid
    1 cc = 1 mL

The same prefixes that were used with meter are used with liter.

Units larger than 1 liter

kiloliter	kL	=	1000 liters
hectoliter	hL	=	100 liters
dekaliter	daL	=	10 liters

Unit equal to 1 liter

liter	L	=	1 liter

Units smaller than 1 liter

deciliter	dL	=	0.1(1/10) liter
centiliter	cL	=	0.01(1/100) liter
milliliter	mL	=	0.001(1/1000) liter

A deciliter is 0.1 ($\frac{1}{10}$) liter.   10 deciliters = 1 liter

A centiliter is 0.01 ($\frac{1}{100}$) liter.   100 centiliters = 1 liter

A milliliter is 0.001 ($\frac{1}{1000}$) liter.   1000 milliliters = 1 liter

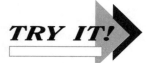

PRACTICE

1. The basic unit of volume in the metric system is the _____. It is the amount of liquid that will fill a cube with a volume of _____ cc.

2. 1 liter = _____ mL

3. 1 mL = _____ cc

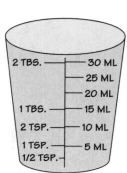

ANSWERS

1. liter, 1000
2. 1000
3. 1

Metric Volume Conversion

After learning the metric units of volume, the next step is to learn how to change from one unit to another. The process is exactly the same as the conversion of metric lengths within the system. Examine the table of most commonly used metric volume equivalents. This information should be memorized.

METRIC VOLUME EQUIVALENTS	
1 mL = 1 cc	The conversion factor is 1.
1 L = 1000 mL	The conversion factor = 1000.
1 L = 1000 cc	The conversion factor = 1000.

There are only two steps in the conversion process:

1. Remember the equivalents. This information provides the conversion factor.
2. Multiply by the conversion factor to convert to smaller units.
    OR
  Divide by the conversion factor to convert to larger units.

A. 2.85 L = _____ mL
  Step 1: Equivalent?
     1 L = 1000 mL   Conversion factor = 1000.
  Step 2: Multiply or Divide?
     The conversion is to a smaller unit. It will take more of the smaller units to make an equivalent amount of the larger units. Multiply by the conversion factor of 1000. Move the decimal point 3 places to the right.
     2.85 L = 2 850 mL

B. 750 mL = _____ L
  Step 1: Equivalent?
     1 L = 1000 mL   Conversion factor = 1000.
  Step 2: Multiply or Divide?
     The conversion is to a larger unit. It will take fewer of the larger unit to make an equivalent amount of smaller units. Divide by the conversion factor of 1000. Move the decimal point 3 places to the left.
     750 mL = 0.75 L

C. _____ cc = 0.85 L
  Step 1: Equivalent?
     1 L = 1000 cc   Conversion factor = 1000.
  Step 2: Multiply or Divide?
     The conversion is to a smaller unit. Multiply by the conversion factor.
     850 cc = 0.85 L

D. _____ mL = 25 cc
  Step 1: Equivalent?
     1 mL = 1 cc
  Step 2: Multiply or Divide?
     The conversion is to the same size unit. The quantity of cubic centimeters will be equal to the quantity of milliliters.
     25 mL = 25 cc

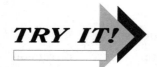

PRACTICE

Convert the metric volume units. Multiply by the conversion factor to change to smaller units. Divide by the conversion factor to change to larger units.

EXAMPLES

3.5 L = _____ mL   (Multiply by the conversion factor to change to smaller units: 3.5 L = 3 500 mL)

620 cc = _____ L   (Divide by the conversion factor to change to larger units: 620 cc = 0.62 L)

8 mL = _____ cc   (Since 1 mL = 1 cc, the quantity of milliliters is the same as the quantity of cubic centimeters: 8 mL = 8 cc)

1. _____ L = 17 mL

2. _____ cc = 5 mL

3. 8.4 L = _____ mL

4. 500 cc = _____ L

ANSWERS

1. 0.017 L   **2.** 5 cc   **3.** 8 400 mL   **4.** 0.5 L

ADDITIONAL PRACTICE

5. 1 cc = _____ mL

6. 7 L = _____ mL

7. 1 mL = _____ L

8. _____ L = 750 mL

9. _____ cc = 3 mL

10. 1500 mL = _____ L

11. 0.5 L = _____ mL

12. 10 mL = _____ L

13. _____ L = 1425 mL

14. 1 mL = _____ cc

15. 2 L = _____ cc

16. _____ mL = 2.7 L

17. _____ mL = 0.85 L

18. 2 cc = _____ mL

19. 10 mL = _____ cc

20. 8.2 L = _____ cc

21. 100 mL = _____ L

22. _____ L = 1000 mL

23. 95 cc = _____ L

24. 15 cc = _____ mL

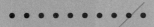

1. The normal daily intake of fluid for an adult is about 1500–2000 milliliters. Express this range in liters.

    ____ L – ____ L

2. The average capacity of an adult urinary bladder is about 500 cc.

    500 cc = ____ mL = ____ L

3. The average adult excretes about 1200–1500 cc of urine every 24 hours. Express this range in milliliters first, then liters.

    1200 cc = ____ mL = ____ L

    1500 cc = ____ mL = ____ L

4. A given syringe holds 3 cc of medication. The capacity of the syringe could also be stated as _____ mL.

5. A certain tuberculin syringe has a capacity of 0.5 mL. What is the volume of this syringe in cubic centimeters (cc)? _____ cc

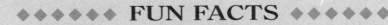

◆ ◆ ◆ ◆ ◆ ◆ **FUN FACTS** ◆ ◆ ◆ ◆ ◆ ◆

The average length of the linen bandages that were used to wrap Egyptian mummies was nearly one kilometer.

PART 5: WEIGHT MEASUREMENT AND CONVERSION

OBJECTIVES

1. *Identify metric units of weight that are larger and smaller than the gram.*
2. *List the most commonly used weight equivalents within the metric system.*
3. *Convert from one weight unit to another within the metric system.*

An overview of eight metric units of weight is presented in this part. However, metric weight conversions are concentrated on the kilogram, gram, milligram, and microgram for application in the medical field.

Weight Measurement

The gram is the basic unit of weight in the metric system. It is the weight of 1 cc or 1 mL of water. A gram is approximately the weight of two paper clips. To express units of weight that are larger and smaller than a gram, the same prefixes are used again. (A kilogram, for reference, is about 2.2 pounds.)

Units larger than 1 gram

kilogram	kg	=	1000 grams
hectogram	hg	=	100 grams
dekagram	dag	=	10 grams

Unit equal to 1 gram

gram	g	=	1 gram

Units smaller than 1 gram

decigram	dg	=	0.1 gram (1/10)
centigram	cg	=	0.01 gram (1/100)
milligram	mg	=	0.001 gram (1/1000)
microgram	mcg, μg	=	0.000001 gram (1/1 000 000)

Notice anything different with the weights?

Another unit which is smaller than a gram (even smaller than a milligram!) and used in drug measurement is the microgram (mcg). Microgram is also symbolized as μg. The microgram is 0.001 milligram, which means 1000 mcg = 1 mg. (That means that 1 μg is one-millionth of a gram!)

A microgram is 0.001 milligram.	
1000 micrograms = 1 milligram	1000 mcg = 1 mg
A milligram is 0.001 gram.	
1000 milligrams = 1 gram	1000 mg = 1 g
A gram is 0.001 kilogram.	
1000 grams = 1 kilogram	1000 g = 1 kg

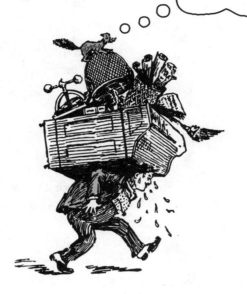

I don't know what he's complaining about. I only weigh 1 gram or 1 cc or 1 mL of water...

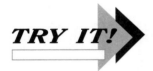

TRY IT!

PRACTICE

1. The basic unit of weight in the metric system is the _____, which is the weight of 1 cc of water. A larger unit of weight is the _____, which is approximately 2.2 pounds. A much smaller unit called the _____ is 0.001 mg.

2. Kilo- means _____ and milli- means _____.

3. 1 kg = _____ g

4. 1000 mg = _____ g

5. 1000 mcg = _____ mg

6. The _____ is symbolized as mcg or μg.

ANSWERS

1. gram; kilogram; microgram
2. 1000; 0.001 (1/1000)
3. 1 kg = 1000 g
4. 1000 mg = 1 g
5. 1000 mcg = 1 mg
6. microgram

Metric Weight Conversion

Conversion between metric weight units is the same process as used with length and volume within the metric system. Examine the most frequently used metric weight equivalents. This information should be memorized.

METRIC WEIGHT EQUIVALENTS	
1 kg = 1000 g	The conversion factor is 1000.
1 g = 1000 mg	The conversion factor is 1000.
1 mg = 1000 mcg	The conversion factor is 1000.

A. 28.5 g = _____ mg
   Step 1: Equivalent?
       1 g = 1000 mg   Conversion factor = 1000.
   Step 2: Multiply or Divide?
       The conversion is to smaller units. Multiply by the conversion factor.
       28.5 g = 28 500 mg

B. _____ kg = 135 g
   Step 1: Equivalent?
       1 kg = 1000 g   Conversion factor = 1000.
   Step 2: Multiply or Divide?
       The conversion is to larger units. Divide by the conversion factor.
       0.135 kg = 135 g

C. _____ g = 4.5 kg
   Step 1: Equivalent?
       1 kg = 1000 g   Conversion factor = 1000.
   Step 2: Multiply or Divide?
       The conversion is to smaller units. Multiply by the conversion factor.
       4 500 g = 4.5 kg

D. 750 mg = _____ g
   Step 1: Equivalent?
       1 g = 1000 mg   Conversion factor = 1000.
   Step 2: Multiply or Divide?
       The conversion is to larger units. Divide by the conversion factor.
       750 mg = 0.75 g

E. _____ mcg = 0.4 mg
    Step 1: Equivalent?
        1 mg = 1000 mcg   Conversion factor = 1000.
    Step 2: Multiply or Divide?
        The conversion is to smaller units. Multiply by the conversion factor.
        400 mcg = 0.4 mg

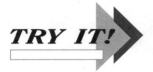

PRACTICE

Convert the metric weight units. Multiply by the conversion factor to change to smaller units. Divide by the conversion factor to change to larger units.

EXAMPLES

    _____ mg = 7.5 g   (Multiply by the conversion factor to convert to a smaller unit. 7 500 mg = 7.5 g)

    180 g = _____ kg   (Divide by the conversion factor to convert to a larger unit. 180 g = 0.18 kg)

---

1. 9.8 kg   = _____ g

2. 0.58 g   = _____ mg

3. _____ g   = 4 mg

4. _____ kg   = 52.8 g

5. _____ mg = 25 mcg

ANSWERS
1. 9800 g
2. 580 mg
3. 0.004 g
4. 0.052 8 kg
5. 0.025 mg

◆◆◆◆◆◆ **FUN FACTS** ◆◆◆◆◆◆

A weight of a caret, the standard unit of measurement for gemstones, is 200 milligrams.

ADDITIONAL PRACTICE

6. 0.75 g = _____ mg   7. _____ g = 0.3 kg

8. 6 250 mg = _____ g   9. _____ kg = 2750 g

10. 8 g = _____ mg   11. _____ mg = 75 mcg

12. 100 mcg = _____ mg   13. 5 mg = _____ g

14. _____ kg = 25 g   15. _____ mg = 19.5 g

16. _____ mcg = 7 mg   17. _____ kg = 150 g

18. 0.05 kg = _____ g   19. _____ g = 4.6 kg

20. 125 mg = _____ g

ON THE JOB

A drug label on a drug container provides pertinent information.

A. Generic and brand name of the drug

B. Dosage strength

C. Expiration date

The dosage strength on the drug label is often called the on-hand dosage or the dosage you have on hand.

Convert the tablet dosage strength as indicated.

1. sulfasalazine   500 mg tablet _____ g

2. triamcinolone   4 mg tablet _____ g

3. codeine sulfate   0.03 g tablet _____ mg

4. morphine sulfate 0.015 g tablet _____ mg

5. The average range of birth weights for newborns is 2900 g–4000 g. Express the range in kilograms.

   _____ kg – _____ kg

6. A premature baby, born before the 37-38 week of gestation, has a birth weight of less than 2.5 kilograms.

   2.5 kg = _____ g

PART 6: CONVERSION BETWEEN SYSTEMS OF MEASUREMENT

OBJECTIVES

1. *Convert between measurements in meters or centimeters and inches.*
2. *Convert between measurements in kilograms and pounds.*

It may sometimes be necessary to convert patient weight and height measurements between systems. The most commonly used conversions are generally accepted *approximations* of equivalence. The units between systems of measurement are *not exact* multiples of one another.

Conversions between Metric and English Systems

> 1 inch (in) = 2.5 centimeters (cm) (The cm is the smaller unit.)
> 1 meter (m) = 39.4 inches (in) (The inch is the smaller unit.)
> 1 kilogram (kg) = 2.2 pounds (lb) (The lb is the smaller unit.)

Convert between units using the conversion factor. Multiply to change to a smaller unit and divide to change to a larger unit.

A. Convert 154 pounds to kilograms.
   Step 1: Equivalent?
      1 kg = 2.2 lb
      The conversion factor is 2.2.
   Step 2: Multiply or Divide?
      The conversion is to a larger unit. Divide by the conversion factor.
      154 ÷ 2.2 = 70
   Step 3: 154 lb = 70 kg

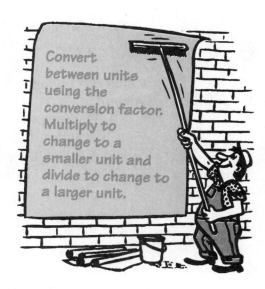

Convert between units using the conversion factor. Multiply to change to a smaller unit and divide to change to a larger unit.

B. Convert 22 inches to centimeters.

   Step 1: Equivalent?

      1 in = 2.5 cm

      The conversion factor is 2.5.

   Step 2: Multiply or Divide?

      The conversion is to a smaller unit. Multiply by the conversion factor.

      22 x 2.5 = 55

   Step 3: 22 in = 55 cm

C. Convert 5 feet 7 inches to centimeters.

   Step 1: 5'7" must be converted to inches before converting to centimeters.

      1 ft = 12 in

      5'7" = (5 x 12) + 7 = 67"

   Step 2: Equivalent?

      1 in = 2.5 cm

      The conversion factor is 2.5.

   Step 3: Multiply or Divide?

      The conversion is to a smaller unit. Multiply by the conversion factor.

      67 x 2.5 = 167.5 cm

   Step 4: 5'7" = 167.5 cm

D. Convert 0.75 meter to inches.

   Step 1: Equivalent?

      1 m = 39.4 in

      The conversion factor is 39.4.

   Step 2: Multiply or Divide?

      The conversion is to a smaller unit. Multiply by the conversion factor.

      0.75 x 39.4 = 29.55

   Step 3: $0.75 \text{ m} \sim 29 \frac{1}{2} \text{ in}$

E. Convert 95 pounds to kilograms. (Round to the nearest whole pound.)

   Step 1: Equivalent?

      1 lb = 2.2 kg

      The conversion factor is 2.2.

   Step 2: Multiply or Divide?

      The conversion is to larger units. Divide by the conversion factor.

      $95 \div 2.2 \sim 43$

   Step 3: $95 \text{ lb} \sim 43 \text{ kg}$

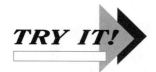

TRY IT!

PRACTICE

1. Change 176 pounds to kilograms. _____

2. Change 40 centimeters to inches. _____

3. Change 6'2" to centimeters. _____

ANSWERS
1. 176 ÷ 2.2 = 80 kg
2. 40 ÷ 2.5 = 16 in
3. 6'2" = (6 x 12) + 2 = 74 in; 74 x 2.5 = 185 cm

ADDITIONAL PRACTICE

Convert the weights to the indicated unit. Express the answer to the nearest whole pound or nearest kilogram.

4. 15.5 kg = _____ lb   5. 99 lb   = _____ kg

6. 30.1 kg = _____ lb   7. 179 lb = _____ kg

8. 100 kg   = _____ lb   9. 15 lb   = _____ kg

Convert the units as indicated. Round to the nearest tenth, if necessary.

10. $5 \frac{1}{2}$ in = _____ cm   11. 4'7"   = _____ cm

12. 25 in   = _____ m   13. 75 in   = _____ m

14. 60 in   = _____ cm   15. 6 ft   = _____ cm

16. 5'5"   = _____ cm

Convert the units as indicated. Round to the nearest whole.

17. 1.75 m = _____ in   18. 85 cm   = _____ in

The weights of three patients were recorded. Convert the units. Round pounds to the nearest whole and kilograms to the nearest tenth, if necessary.

1. 196 pounds   =   _____ kg

2. 157 pounds   =   _____ kg

3. 61 kilograms =   _____ lb

The heights of four patients were recorded. Convert the units. (Round to the nearest whole, if necessary.)

4. 1.8 m   =   _____ in

5. 157.5 cm   =   _____ in

6. 72 in   =   _____ cm

7. 5'11"   =   _____ cm

◆◆◆◆◆◆ FUN FACTS ◆◆◆◆◆◆

The average weight of children born in May is approximately 200 grams heavier than that of children born in other months.

PART 7: FAHRENHEIT AND CELSIUS TEMPERATURE CONVERSION

OBJECTIVES

1. *Convert Fahrenheit temperatures to degrees Celsius.*
2. *Convert Celsius temperatures to degrees Fahrenheit.*

Temperature can be measured in degrees Fahrenheit or degrees Celsius. Because of the difference in the Fahrenheit and Celsius scales, a Celsius temperature will always be fewer degrees than its equivalent number of degrees Fahrenheit.

Fahrenheit and Celsius Thermometers

Notice the difference in the scales of the two thermometers.

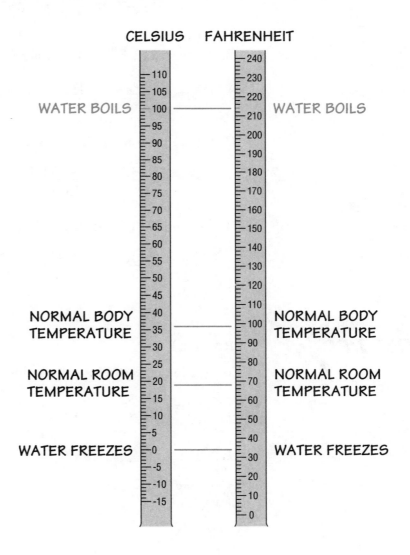

Conversion from Fahrenheit to Celsius

Follow a two-step procedure to convert from Fahrenheit to Celsius. These two steps *must* be done in order! (Remember that a Celsius temperature is fewer degrees than its equivalent Fahrenheit temperature.)

1. Subtract 32 from the Fahrenheit degrees.
2. Divide by 1.8.

The result is degrees Celsius.

$$C = \frac{F - 32}{1.8}$$

A. Convert 32°F (freezing point of water) to degrees Celsius.

$$C = \frac{32 - 32}{1.8} = \frac{0}{1.8} = 0°C$$

B. Convert 212°F (boiling point of water) to degrees Celsius.

$$C = \frac{212 - 32}{1.8} = \frac{180}{1.8} = 100°C$$

C. Convert 4°F to degrees Celsius (rounded to the nearest tenth).

$$C = \frac{F - 32}{1.8} = \frac{4 - 32}{1.8} = \frac{-28}{1.8} \sim -15.6°C$$

D. Convert 60°F to degrees Celsius (rounded to the nearest tenth).

$$C = \frac{F - 32}{1.8} = \frac{60 - 32}{1.8} = \frac{28}{1.8} \sim 15.6°C$$

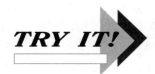

TRY IT!

PRACTICE

Convert to degrees Celsius. Round to the nearest tenth.

$$C = \frac{F - 32}{1.8}$$

1. 1°F _____ °C

2. 105°F _____ °C

ANSWERS
1. -17.2°C
2. 40.6°C

Conversion from Celsius to Fahrenheit

Follow a two-step procedure to convert from Celsius to Fahrenheit. These two steps *must* be done in order!

1. Multiply 1.8 times degrees Celsius.
2. Add 32.

The result is degrees Fahrenheit.

$$F = 1.8\ C + 32$$

A. Convert 20°C (room temperature) to degrees Fahrenheit.

$$F = (1.8)(20) + 32 = 36 + 32 = 68°F$$

B. Convert 37°C (normal body temperature) to degrees Fahrenheit.

$$
\begin{aligned}
F &= 1.8\ C + 32 \\
&= 1.8\ (37) + 32 \\
&= 66.6 + 32 \\
&= 98.6°F
\end{aligned}
$$

C. Convert 15°C to degrees Fahrenheit.

$$
\begin{aligned}
F &= 1.8\ C + 32 \\
&= 1.8\ (15) + 32 \\
&= 27 + 32 \\
&= 59°F
\end{aligned}
$$

D. Convert 57°C to degrees Fahrenheit.

$$
\begin{aligned}
F &= 1.8\ C + 32 \\
&= 102.6 + 32 \\
&= 134.6°F
\end{aligned}
$$

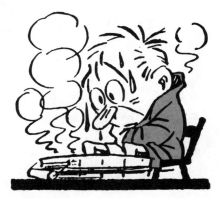

If 37° Celsius is normal body temperature, then why don't I feel like 98.6° Fahrenheit?

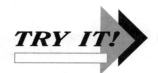
TRY IT!

PRACTICE

Convert to degrees Fahrenheit. (Round to the nearest tenth.)

$$F = 1.8 C + 32$$

1. 26.5°C _____ °F

2. 41°C _____ °F

ANSWERS
1. 79.7°F
2. 105.8°F

ADDITIONAL PRACTICE

Convert the temperatures to degrees Fahrenheit.

3. 25°C = _____ °F

4. 45°C = _____ °F

5. 3°C = _____ °F

6. 10°C = _____ °F

7. 38.5°C = _____ °F

Convert the temperatures to degrees Celsius. Round to the nearest tenth.

8. 0°F = _____ °C

9. 35°F = _____ °C

10. 75°F = _____ °C

11. 6°F = _____ °C

12. 100°F = _____ °C

Normal body temperature depends upon the method used to obtain the measurement. Convert the Fahrenheit temperatures to Celsius and round to the nearest tenth, if necessary.

1. A temperature taken by placing the thermometer in the rectum is a rectal temperature. This method is usually used for infants and children and always used for unconscious patients. Normal rectal temperature is 99.6°F.

   99.6°F   =   _____ °C

2. A temperature taken by placing the thermometer in the mouth is an oral temperature. Normal oral temperature is 98.6°F.

   98.6°F   =   _____ °C

3. A temperature taken by placing the thermometer in the armpit is an axillary temperature. Normal axillary temperature is 97.6°F.

   97.6°F   =   _____ °C

4. A temperature over 38°C is considered to be a fever.

   38°C   =   _____ °F

5. Most disease-causing bacteria grow best at a temperature of approximately 37°C.

   37°C   =   _____ °F

UNIT 3 REVIEW

EXERCISES

Identify each metric unit as a WEIGHT, VOLUME, or LENGTH measurement. Then print the metric symbol for each unit.

1. kilogram _____ _____

2. meter _____ _____

3. millimeter _____ _____

4. cubic centimeter _____ _____

5. centimeter _____ _____

6. milligram _____ _____

7. liter _____ _____

8. microgram _____ _____

9. millimeter _____ _____

10. gram _____ _____

Interpret each metric symbol.

11. mL _____

12. kg _____

13. mm _____

14. μg _____

15. cc _____

16. mcg _____

17. cm _____

18. mg _____

19. L _____

20. g _____

Write each metric measure in correct symbolic notation.

21. $\frac{1}{2}$ milliliter _____

22. 1,225 micrograms _____

23. 1 $\frac{40}{100}$ grams _____

24. 2 $\frac{1}{4}$ cubic centimeters _____

25. $\frac{3}{4}$ milligram _____

26. $\frac{8}{100}$ meter _____

27. ten and four-tenths kilograms _____

28. seven liters _____

29. three hundredths of a milligram _____

30. sixty-hundredths of a cubic centimeter _____

Fill in the blank to express the equivalent or the generally accepted (approximate) equivalent.

31. _____ mL = 1 cc   32. _____ in = 1 m   33. _____ cm = 1 in

34. _____ g = 1 kg   35. _____ mcg = 1 mg   36. _____ mg = 1 g

37. _____ cm = 1 m   38. _____ mL = 1 L   39. _____ mm = 1 m

40. _____ lb = 1 kg   41. _____ cc = 1 L   42. _____ m = 1 km

43. _____ mm = 1 cm   44. _____ μg = 1 mg   45. _____ cc = 1 mL

Convert the metric length.

46. 6.3 m = _____ cm   47. 176 mm = _____ cm   48. _____ m = 600 mm

49. 0.4 km = _____ m   50. 6 mm = _____ cm   51. _____ m = 45 cm

52. 1.5 km = _____ m   53. _____ mm = 8.25 cm   54. _____ km = 95 m

55. 160.5 cm = _____ m

Convert the metric volume.

56. _____ mL = 4.5 L   57. _____ L = 3500 cc   58. 0.75 mL = _____ cc

59. 1.5 cc = _____ mL   60. 3 mL = _____ cc   61. 125 mL = _____ L

62. 2.7 cc = _____ mL   63. _____ L = 125 mL   64. 8 mL = _____ cc

65. _____ cc = 0.7 L

Convert the metric weight.

66. 4.25 kg = _____ g   67. 0.05 g = _____ mg   68. _____ mg = 25 mcg

69. 150 g = _____ kg   70. 0.4 mg = _____ g   71. _____ mcg = 2 mg

72. _____ kg = 4200 g   73. _____ g = 100 mg   74. _____ mg = 50 mcg

75. _____ mg = 1.3 g

Convert the temperatures as indicated. Round to the nearest tenth, when necessary.

76. 103°F   = ____ °C   **77.** 25.5°C   = ____ °F   **78.** 96°F   = ____ °C

79. 35°C   = ____ °F   **80.** 32°F   = ____ °C   **81.** 26.7°C   = ____ °F

82. 93.5°F   = ____ °C   **83.** 48°C   = ____ °F   **84.** 76°F   = ____ °C

85. 100°C   = ____ °F   **86.** 38.9°C   = ____ °F   **87.** 212°F   = ____ °C

88. 20°C   = ____ °F   **89.** 43°C   = ____ °F   **90.** 100°F   = ____ °C

Convert from one system of measurement to another. Round to the nearest tenth, if necessary.

91. 57.7 kg   = ____ lb   **92.** 7 in   = ____ cm   **93.** 97 lb   = ____ kg

94. 58 cm   = ____ in   **95.** 74 in   = ____ m   **96.** 44 kg   = ____ lb

97. 4'7"   = ____ cm   **98.** 4.5 cm   = ____ in   **99.** 5'6"   = ____ cm

100. 18 lb   = ____ kg

ON THE JOB

The average length of a newborn is about 50 cm.

1. 50 cm   =   ____ mm

2. 50 cm   =   ____ m

The heights of four patients were recorded. Express the measurement in the indicated unit. Round to the nearest hundredth, if necessary.

3. Patient Agnes: 180 cm   = ____ m

4. Patient Brendan: 192.5 cm   = ____ m

5. Patient Eddie: 1.7 m   = ____ cm

6. Patient Flo: 1.85 m   = ____ cm

The patient's wrist measurements were recorded.

7. Left wrist: 15.4 cm   = ____ mm

8. Right wrist: 16.3 cm   = ____ mm

During a physical assessment, two moles on a patient's back were noted and measured.

9. Mole A: 17 mm   =   _____ cm

10. Mole B: 9 mm   =   _____ cm

11. A child was admitted to the emergency room with a cut which was noted in the records.

    Cut: 125 mm   =   _____ cm

12. The adult gallbladder has the capacity for about 50 cc of bile.

    50 cc   =   _____ mL

13. A given tuberculin syringe holds 1 cc. The capacity of this syringe is _____ mL.

14. A prefilled syringe has a capacity of 2.5 mL. What is the volume of this syringe in cubic centimeters (cc)? _____

15. Oliguria is a condition in which urination is diminished to between 100 and 400 mL in 24 hours. Express the range in cubic centimeters. _____ cc – _____ cc

16. Anuria is a condition in which there is an absence or suppression of urine, characterized by excretion of less than 100 mL urine in 24 hours.

    100 mL   =   _____ cc

A drug label on a drug container provides pertinent information.

A. Generic and brand name of the drug

B. Dosage strength

C. Expiration date

The dosage strength on the drug label is often called the on-hand dosage or the dosage you have on hand.

Convert the tablet dosage strength as indicated to grams.

17. neomycin sulfate   500 mg tablet   _____ g

18. ibuprofen   600 mg tablet   _____ g

19. penicillin   125 mg tablet   _____ g

Convert the tablet dosage strength to milligrams.

20. acetylsalicylic acid   0.3 g tablet   _____ mg

21. sodium bicarbonate 0.32 g tablet   _____ mg

22. phenobarbital   0.06 g tablet   _____ mg

23. The average birth weight of a newborn is about 3.3 kg.

    3.3 kg   =   _____ g

24. The fetus in the fourth month of development weighs about 286 grams.

    286 g   =   _____ kg

25. The fetus in the sixth month of development weighs about 908 g.

    908 g   =   _____ kg

The weights of three patients were recorded. Convert the units. (Round pounds to the nearest whole and kilograms to the nearest tenth, if necessary.)

26. Patient Kendra: 75 kg   =   _____ lb

27. Patient Larry: 122 lb   =   _____ kg

28. Patient Rene: 147 lb   =   _____ kg

The heights of three patients were recorded. Convert the units. (Round to the nearest whole, if necessary.)

29. Patient Henry: 1.7 m   =   _____ in

30. Patient Nick: 177.8 cm   =   _____ in

31. Patient Owen: 65 in   =   _____ cm

32. The most desirable temperature for a weighing room for babies is approximately 24.5°C.

    24.5°C   =   _____ °F

33. The temperature of bath water for an adult should be about 110°F.

    110°F   =   _____ °C
    (Round to the nearest tenth.)

34. The temperature of bath water for a baby should not be as warm as that for an adult. A baby's bath should be approximately 95°F.

$$95°F \quad = \quad \underline{\hspace{2cm}} °C$$

35. The temperature of the room where baths are given should be approximately 23.9°C–26.7°C. Express the range in degrees Fahrenheit and round the temperatures to the nearest whole degree. _____ °F – _____ °F

36. The room temperature is 21°C. Express this temperature in degrees Fahrenheit, rounded to the nearest whole degree.

$$21°C \quad = \quad \underline{\hspace{2cm}} °F$$

◆◆◆◆◆◆ **FUN FACTS** ◆◆◆◆◆◆

An average hummingbird has a body temperature of 111°F and beats its wings at a rate of approximately 75 times per minute.

UNIT 4

Percent, Ratio, and Proportion

PART 1: PERCENT

OBJECTIVES

1. *Understand the meaning of percent.*
2. *Express percents as equivalent decimals.*
3. *Express percents as equivalent fractions.*
4. *Understand solution strength stated as a percent.*

Percents are used frequently in everyday life. In this discussion, the presentation is directed toward the use of percent relating to solution strength and dosage calculation.

The Meaning of Percent

Percent is another kind of fraction that always has a denominator of 100. So far we have discussed common fractions and decimals which are two other kinds of fractions. Percent means "per 100" or "÷ 100." Remember that the fraction bar means "divided by."

6%	=	6 percent	=	6 per 100	=	$\frac{6}{100}$
25%	=	25 percent	=	25 per 100	=	$\frac{25}{100}$
100%	=	100 percent	=	100 per 100	=	$\frac{100}{100}$

Dividing by 100 results in "hundredths" as can be seen. Another way of saying percent is hundredths.

1%	=	1 percent	=	$\frac{1}{100}$	=	1 hundredth
50%	=	50 percent	=	$\frac{50}{100}$	=	50 hundredths
75%	=	75 percent	=	$\frac{75}{100}$	=	75 hundredths

Percent can be thought of as:

hundredths	(20% = 20 hundredths = 0.20)
per 100	(20% = 20 per 100)
divided by 100	(20% = $\frac{20}{100}$)
out of 100	(20% = 20 out of 100)

Common fractions can be equal to one ($\frac{7}{7}$), less than one ($\frac{3}{7}$), and greater than one ($\frac{15}{7}$). Decimals can represent one (1), less than one (0.5), and more than one (1.5). Percents, too, can be equal to one (100% = $\frac{100}{100}$), less than one (30% = $\frac{30}{100}$), and greater than one (150% = $\frac{150}{100}$).

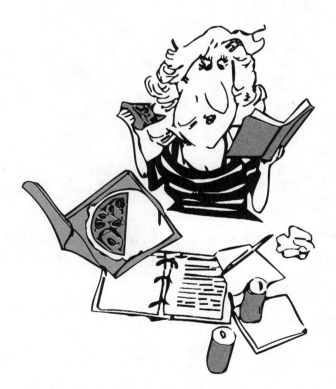

"Any way you slice it, I've eaten 50% or 50 percent or 50/100 of this 6-slice pizza."

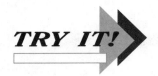

TRY IT!

PRACTICE

Fill in the blanks.

1. Percent is a kind of fraction that always has a denominator of _____.

2. Percent means hundredths, per _____, and divided by _____.

EXAMPLE						
	175%	=	$\frac{175}{100}$	=	175 ÷ 100	= 175 hundredths

3.   35% = _____ = _____ = _____

4.   100% = _____ = _____ = _____

5.   125% = _____ = _____ = _____

6.   3% = _____ = _____ = _____

ANSWERS

1. 100

2. 100, 100

3. $\frac{35}{100}$, 35 ÷ 100, 35 hundredths

4. $\frac{100}{100}$, 100 ÷ 100, 100 hundredths

5. $\frac{125}{100}$, 125 ÷ 100, 125 hundredths

6. $\frac{3}{100}$, 3 ÷ 100, 3 hundredths

Expressing Percents as Equivalent Decimals

The denominator of a percent is always 100. It is not difficult to find the equivalent decimal, for example, 45% = $\frac{45}{100}$, 45 ÷ 100 = 0.45.

4%	=	$\frac{4}{100}$	=	0.04
35%	=	$\frac{35}{100}$	=	0.35
100%	=	$\frac{100}{100}$	=	1.
125%	=	$\frac{125}{100}$	=	1.25

To convert percent to a decimal, drop the percent sign and divide by 100. Move the decimal point two places to the left.

5%	5.	0.05		
95%	95.	0.95		
150%	150.	1.50	=	1.5

Use *extreme* care when handling percentages with fractions such as $\frac{1}{4}$%, $\frac{1}{2}$%, or $16\frac{3}{4}$ %. Express the common fraction as a decimal fraction *first*. Only then, change the percent to a decimal.

$12\frac{1}{2}$ %	=	12.5%	⟶	12.5	⟶	0.125
$\frac{1}{4}$ %	=	0.25%	⟶	0.25	⟶	0.0025
$\frac{1}{2}$ %	=	0.5%	⟶	0.5	⟶	0.005
$\frac{3}{4}$ %	=	0.75%	⟶	0.75	⟶	0.0075

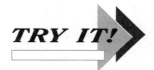
TRY IT!

EXAMPLES

$\frac{1}{10}$ %	=	0.1%	=	0.1	=	0.001
85%	=	85%	=	85.	=	0.85
175%	=	175%	=	175.	=	1.75

PRACTICE

1. 100% _____   _____   _____

2. $\frac{3}{4}$ % _____   _____   _____

3. 30% _____   _____   _____

4. 95% _____   _____   _____

5. 110% _____   _____   _____

ANSWERS

1. 1
2. 0.0075
3. 0.30
4. 0.95
5. 1.10

Expressing Percents as Equivalent Fractions

Remember that percent means "hundredths" and "per 100" and "divided by 100."

To change a percent to a fraction, first express the percent as a fraction with a denominator of 100. Then divide to reduce that fraction to lowest terms.

$$25\% = \frac{25}{100} = \frac{1}{4}$$

$$50\% = \frac{50}{100} = \frac{1}{2}$$

$$75\% = \frac{75}{100} = \frac{3}{4}$$

$$100\% = \frac{100}{100} = 1$$

$$125\% = \frac{125}{100} = 1\frac{25}{100} = 1\frac{1}{4}$$

When dealing with fractional percents or percents with fractions, recall complex fractions. Remember that the fraction bar means "divided by."

A. $\frac{1}{2}\% = \frac{1}{2}$ per 100 $= \dfrac{\frac{1}{2}}{100} = \frac{1}{2} \div \frac{100}{1} = \frac{1}{2} \times \frac{1}{100} = \frac{1}{200}$

B. $33\frac{1}{3}\% = 33\frac{1}{3}$ per 100 $=$

$$\dfrac{33\frac{1}{3}}{100} = \frac{100}{3} \div \frac{100}{1} = \frac{100}{3} \times \frac{1}{100} = \frac{1}{3}$$

C. $66\frac{2}{3}\% = 66\frac{2}{3}$ per 100 $=$

$$\dfrac{66\frac{2}{3}}{100} = \frac{200}{3} \div \frac{100}{1} = \frac{200}{3} \times \frac{1}{100} = \frac{2}{3}$$

D. $0.25\% = 0.25$ per 100 $=$

$$\dfrac{\frac{25}{100}}{100} = \frac{25}{100} \div \frac{100}{1} = \frac{25}{100} \times \frac{1}{100} = \frac{25}{10000} = \frac{1}{400}$$

Less than 100% is less than one whole. More than 100% is more than one whole. 100% is one whole thing.

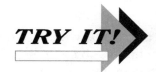
TRY IT!

PRACTICE

Express each percent as a common fraction in lowest terms.

EXAMPLE

$$30\% \quad = \quad 30 \text{ per } 100 \quad = \quad \frac{30}{100} \quad = \quad \frac{3}{10}$$

1. 55% = ___ per ____ = —— = ——

2. 60% = ___ per ____ = —— = ——

3. $\frac{1}{4}\%$ = ___ per ____ = —— = ——

4. $37\frac{1}{2}\%$ = ___ per ____ = —— = ——

5. 0.75% = ___ per ____ = —— = ——

ANSWERS

1. $55 \text{ per } 100 = \frac{55}{100} = \frac{11}{20}$

2. $60 \text{ per } 100 = \frac{60}{100} = \frac{3}{5}$

3. $\frac{1}{4} \text{ per } 100 = \frac{\frac{1}{4}}{100} = \frac{1}{400}$

4. $37\frac{1}{2} \text{ per } 100 = \frac{37\frac{1}{2}}{100} = \frac{75}{200} = \frac{3}{8}$

5. $0.75 \text{ per } 100 = \frac{\frac{3}{4}}{100} = \frac{3}{400}$

Solution Strength as Percent

Percent may be used to state the strength of a solution. A solution is a preparation in which one or more substances have been dissolved in liquid. Liquid is added to a substance to reach a required strength.

Percent strength describes the amount of substance that was dissolved in a liquid to form the solution.

A. A 10% drug solution means that there are 10 parts of pure drug in 100 parts of solution.

B. A $2\frac{1}{2}\%$ drug solution means that there are $2\frac{1}{2}$ parts of pure drug in 100 parts of solution.

Any solution is made up of a solute and a solvent. The **solute** is the substance which is dissolved in liquid to form the solution. The **solvent** is the liquid which is added to the solute to form the solution.

If the solute is in dry form, it is measured in grams (by weight). If the solute is in liquid form, it is measured in milliliters (by volume). The total volume of a solution (solute and solvent combined) is measured in milliliters.

C. 1% solution = 1 g/100 mL

A 1% solution means that 1 gram of pure drug (dry form) was dissolved in enough liquid to make 100 milliliters of solution.

D. 1% solution = 1 mL/100 mL

A 1% solution means that 1 milliliter of pure drug (liquid form) was dissolved in enough liquid to form 100 milliliters of solution.

E. 4% solution = $\frac{4}{100}$ = $\frac{2}{50}$ = $\frac{1}{25}$

A 4% strength is obtained by dissolving 4 mL (or 4 g) of pure solute in enough liquid to form 100 mL of solution. It is the same strength that is obtained by dissolving 2 mL (or 2 g) of pure solute in enough liquid to form 50 mL of solution; 1 mL (or 1 g) of pure solute in 25 mL of solution also has a 4% strength.

F. Solution strength in percent

Five grams of pure solute in 25 mL of solution is equivalent to the fraction $\frac{5}{25}$. To express a solution strength in percent, the fraction must be stated per 100 mL of solution. So $\frac{5}{25} = \frac{?}{100}$ or $\frac{5}{25}$ is equivalent to $\frac{20}{100}$, which is another way of saying 20%.

Therefore, 5 g of pure solute in 25 mL of solution is a 20% solution.

Solution strength stated in percent means:
grams of pure solute (dry form) per 100 milliliters of solution

OR

milliliters of pure solute (liquid form) per 100 milliliters of solution

If the solute is in dry form, it is measured in grams (by weight). If the solute is in liquid form, it is measured in milliliters (by volume).

What's a solute?

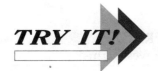
TRY IT!

PRACTICE

1. A 5% solution made with pure drug (liquid form) means 5 _____ of pure drug in 100 _____ of solution.
2. A 5% solution made with pure drug (dry form) means 5 _____ of pure drug in 100 _____ of solution.
3. A 5% solution could by made by dissolving 5 grams of pure drug in enough liquid to make _____ milliliters of solution. A 5% solution could also be made by dissolving 1 gram of pure drug in enough liquid to make _____ milliliters of solution.

ANSWERS
1. milliliters, milliliters
2. grams, milliliters
3. 100 mL, 20 mL

ADDITIONAL PRACTICE
Express each percent as an equivalent decimal.

PERCENT	DECIMAL
4. 100%	_____
5. 5%	_____
6. 76%	_____
7. 0.5%	_____
8. 150%	_____
9. 8%	_____
10. $62\frac{1}{2}$%	_____
11. $\frac{1}{2}$%	_____
12. 200%	_____
13. 10%	_____
14. 50%	_____
15. 3.2%	_____
16. $\frac{3}{4}$%	_____
17. 18.25%	_____
18. 0.03%	_____

	PERCENT	FRACTION (denominator 100)	FRACTION (lowest terms)
19.	16%	_____	_____
20.	4%	_____	_____
21.	$\frac{1}{2}$ %	_____	_____
22.	$66\frac{2}{3}$ %	_____	_____
23.	25%	_____	_____
24.	80%	_____	_____
25.	75%	_____	_____
26.	0.05%	_____	_____
27.	$33\frac{1}{3}$ %	_____	_____
28.	400%	_____	_____
29.	60%	_____	_____
30.	3%	_____	_____
31.	35%	_____	_____
32.	130%	_____	_____
33.	100%	_____	_____

◆◆◆◆◆◆ **FUN FACTS** ◆◆◆◆◆◆

The head of a newborn baby makes up about 25% of its total weight.

A 5% glucose solution has been prepared.

    1. How many grams of glucose are in 100 mL of solution? _____

    2. How many grams of glucose are in 20 mL of solution? _____

A 10% drug solution is in the supply cabinet.

    3. How many grams of the drug are contained in 100 mL of this solution? _____

    4. How many grams of the drug are contained in 20 mL of this solution? _____

    5. How many grams of the drug are contained in 10 mL of this solution? _____

The drug label states that 25 mL of pure drug are contained in 100 mL of solution.

    6. What is the strength of the solution in percent? _____

    7. How many milliliters of pure drug are contained in 4 mL of solution? _____

    8. How many milliliters of pure drug are contained in 200 mL of solution? _____

Five grams of pure solute are contained in 10 mL of solution.

    9. What is the strength of the solution in percent? _____

    10. How many grams of pure solute are contained in 100 mL of solution? _____

PART 2: DECIMALS AND FRACTIONS AS EQUIVALENT PERCENTS

OBJECTIVES

1. *Express decimals as equivalent percents.*
2. *Express fractions as equivalent percents.*

There are times in everyday situations when information that is given in decimal or fraction form is better understood in its equivalent percent form. Changing decimals and fractions to percents is the reverse of the processes that were presented in Unit 4, Part 1.

Changing Decimals to Percents

Remember that a percent is changed to an equivalent decimal by dropping the percent sign and dividing by 100 ($\frac{1}{2}$ % = 0.5% = 0.005, 3% = 0.03, or 16% = 0.16). In the reverse, a decimal may be expressed as a percent. **To convert a decimal to a percent, multiply by 100.** Move the decimal point two places to the right and add a percent sign.

0.125	=	12.5%
3.9	=	390%
0.75	=	75%

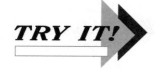

PRACTICE

Express each decimal as an equivalent percent.

EXAMPLES

0.50	=	50%
2.34	=	234%
0.005	=	0.5%

1. 0.05   =   _____%

2. 0.25   =   _____%

3. 0.345   =   _____%

4. 1.75   =   _____%

5. 0.01   =   _____%

ANSWERS

1. 5%
2. 25%
3. 34.5%
4. 175%
5. 1%

Changing Fractions to Percents

A common fraction is converted to a percent in two steps:

Step 1. Express the fraction as a decimal. (Divide the numerator by the denominator.)

Step 2. Change the decimal to a percent by multiplying by 100.

$$\frac{1}{4} = 1 \div 4 = 0.25 = 25\%$$

$$\frac{3}{8} = 3 \div 8 = 0.375 = 37.5\%$$

$$\frac{2}{5} = 2 \div 5 = 0.4 = 40\%$$

$$1\frac{3}{4} = \frac{7}{4} = 7 \div 4 = 1.75 = 175\%$$

Rounding may be sometimes necessary when changing common fractions to percents.

A. Round to the nearest tenth percent. Notice that the division must be carried out four places to the right of the decimal point to round to the nearest percent.

$$\frac{4}{7} = 4 \div 7 \sim 0.5714... \sim 57.1\%$$

$$\frac{7}{6} = 7 \div 6 \sim 1.1666 ... \sim 116.7\%$$

B. Round to the nearest whole percent. Notice that the division must be carried out three places to the right of the decimal point to round to the nearest whole percent.

$$\frac{5}{12} = 5 \div 12 \sim 0.416... \sim 42\%$$

$$\frac{5}{6} = 5 \div 6 \sim 0.833... \sim 83\%$$

$$1\frac{5}{6} = \frac{11}{6} = 11 \div 6 \sim 1.833... \sim 183\%$$

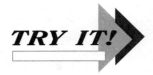

TRY IT!

PRACTICE

Change the common fraction to its equivalent percent.

1. $\frac{1}{2}$ = ____%

2. $\frac{5}{8}$ = ____%

3. $\frac{3}{4}$ = ____%

Change the common fraction to its equivalent percent, rounded to the nearest tenth percent.

4. $\frac{1}{9}$ = _____%

5. $\frac{4}{11}$ = _____%

ANSWERS

1. $0.5 = 50\%$
2. $0.625 = 62.5\%$
3. $0.75 = 75\%$
4. $0.1111... \sim 11.1\%$
5. $0.3636... \sim 36.4\%$

ADDITIONAL PRACTICE

Express each decimal as an equivalent percent.

DECIMAL	PERCENT
6. 0.2	_____
7. 0.892	_____
8. 0.055	_____
9. 6.75	_____
10. 0.08	_____
11. 0.01	_____
12. 1.08	_____
13. 0.001	_____
14. 1.45	_____
15. 0.30	_____
16. 0.15	_____
17. 0.5	_____
18. 0.45	_____
19. 3.5	_____
20. 0.07	_____

Express each common fraction as a percent. (Round to the nearest tenth percent if necessary.)

	COMMON FRACTION	DECIMAL	PERCENT
21.	$\frac{4}{8}$	_____	_____
22.	$\frac{28}{7}$	_____	_____
23.	$\frac{7}{8}$	_____	_____
24.	$\frac{3}{5}$	_____	_____
25.	$\frac{2}{3}$	_____	_____
26.	$2\frac{1}{8}$	_____	_____
27.	$\frac{17}{20}$	_____	_____
28.	$\frac{5}{10}$	_____	_____
29.	$1\frac{1}{5}$	_____	_____
30.	$\frac{9}{12}$	_____	_____
31.	$2\frac{1}{4}$	_____	_____
32.	$3\frac{1}{2}$	_____	_____
33.	$\frac{3}{4}$	_____	_____
34.	$\frac{5}{8}$	_____	_____
35.	$\frac{10}{5}$	_____	_____

ON THE JOB

• • • • • • • • • •

Express the following patient information in percent. Round to the nearest tenth percent, if necessary.

1. 1 out of 45 patients received insulin. _____%
2. 75 out of 125 patients required follow-up visits. _____%
3. 1 out of 110 patients received a blood transfusion. _____%
4. Nearly 0.07 of the patients stayed fewer than two days. _____%
5. Only 0.005 of the patients remained in the hospital for more than two weeks. _____%

OBJECTIVES

1. *Compare quantities using ratios.*
2. *Express ratios as equivalent fractions, decimals, and percents.*
3. *Express ratios in lowest terms.*
4. *Identify a ratio that expresses a rate.*
5. *Determine the unknown term in a ratio with an implied component.*
6. *Understand solution strength stated as a ratio.*

Data are often presented in the form of a ratio. A ratio can be used to make a comparison that shows the relationship between two like quantities or it can be used to express a rate, when the quantities have different labels.

Introduction to Ratios

A ratio is a comparison between two quantities or the relationship of one quantity to another. The two terms of a ratio are separated by a colon. The colon is read "to."

For example,
   3 : 5 is read 3 to 5
   1 : 4 is read 1 to 4

The ratio (1 : 4) is another expression that is equivalent to a fraction ($\frac{1}{4}$), a decimal (0.25), and a percent (25%). Similarly, $3 : 5 = \frac{3}{5} = 0.6 = 60\%$.

A ratio is often stated in fractional form. The terms of the ratio become the terms of the fraction (numerator and denominator). The fraction bar means "divided by" so a ratio is an expression of division.

$$1 : 2 = 1 \text{ to } 2 = \frac{1}{2} = 1 \div 2$$

$$4 : 3 = 4 \text{ to } 3 = \frac{4}{3} = 4 \div 3$$

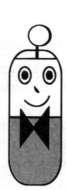

1 gram per capsule is a ratio of 1 : 1.
It means 1 g : 1 capsule.
The implied term in the ratio is the number 1.

Just like fractions, a ratio can be expressed in lowest terms.

$$10 : 12 = 10 \text{ to } 12 = \frac{10}{12} \qquad \frac{10}{12} = \frac{5}{6} = 5 \text{ to } 6 = 5 : 6$$

10 : 12 is equivalent to 5 : 6.   5 : 6 is lowest terms.

$$4 : 6 = 4 \text{ to } 6 = \frac{4}{6} \qquad \frac{4}{6} = \frac{2}{3} = 2 \text{ to } 3 = 2 : 3$$

4 : 6 is equivalent to 2 : 3.   2 : 3 is lowest terms.

The following picture illustrates several ratios, or comparisons. Notice that the labels (shaded squares, unshaded squares, total squares) are *critical* for the correct meaning of the ratio.

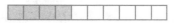

A. There are 4 shaded squares compared to 10 total squares.
   4 : 10 (or 2 : 5)
   4 shaded squares : 10 total squares = 4 : 10 (or 2 : 5)

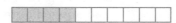

B. There are 6 unshaded squares compared to 10 total squares.
   6 : 10 (or 3 : 5)
   6 unshaded squares : 10 total squares = 6 : 10 (or 3 : 5)

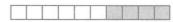

C. There are 4 shaded squares compared to 6 unshaded squares.
   4 : 6 (or 2 : 3).
   4 shaded squares : 6 unshaded squares = 4 : 6 (or 2 : 3)

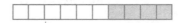

D. There are 6 unshaded squares compared to 4 shaded squares.
   6 : 4 (or 3 : 2).
   6 unshaded squares: 4 shaded squares = 6 : 4 (or 3 : 2)

Ratios Using Like and Unlike Measurements

A ratio can compare like measurements or unlike measurements. Observe the labels very carefully! When like measurements are compared, the labels are similar. When the labels of the numbers are not similar, the ratio is considered to be a rate.

Like Measurements:

4 *male patients* compared to 25 *total patients* $4 : 25 \left(\frac{4}{25}\right)$

4 *male patients* compared to 21 *female patients* $4 : 21 \left(\frac{4}{21}\right)$

5 *red apples* compared to 8 *total apples* $5 : 8 \left(\frac{5}{8}\right)$

5 *red apples* compared to 3 *green apples* $5 : 3 \left(\frac{5}{3}\right)$

Unlike Measurements:

3 *apples* for (compared to) 79 *cents* $3 : 79 \left(\frac{3}{79}\right)$

10 *mg* in (compared to) 2 *tablets* $10 : 2 \left(\frac{10}{2}\right)$

82 *miles* per (compared to) 3 *hours* $82 : 3 \left(\frac{82}{3}\right)$

3 *dollars* per (compared to) 2 *pounds* $3 : 2 \left(\frac{3}{2}\right)$

2 *tablets* every (compared to) 9 *hours* $2 : 9 \left(\frac{2}{9}\right)$

3 *mg* in (compared to) 10 *mL* $3 : 10 \left(\frac{3}{10}\right)$

Remember when a ratio is used to express a rate, the quantities in the ratio have different labels.

Implied Term in a Ratio

In many real life situations, a term in a ratio is implied (not stated directly). Here are some examples:

55 miles per hour is a ratio of 55 : 1. It means 55 miles : 1 hour.
The implied term in the ratio is the number 1.

8 times faster is a ratio of 8 : 1.
The implied term in the ratio is the number 1.

10 mg per milliliter is a ratio of 10 : 1. It means 10 mg : 1 mL.
The implied term in the ratio is the number 1.

250 mg per tablet is a ratio of 250 : 1. It means 250 mg : 1 tablet.
The implied term in the ratio is the number 1.

1 gram per capsule is a ratio of 1 : 1. It means 1 g : 1 capsule.
The implied term in the ratio is the number 1.

3 times farther is a ratio of 3 : 1.
The implied term in the ratio is the number 1.

2 dollars per dozen is the ratio of 2 : 1. It means 2 dollars : 1 dozen.
The implied term in the ratio is the number 1.

Fractional Term in a Ratio

A ratio may have a fraction as one of its terms. An equivalent ratio with whole numbers is easier to use.

Suppose $\frac{1}{2}$ pound costs 49¢. The ratio is $\frac{1}{2}$: 49 or $\frac{\frac{1}{2}}{49}$.

(Remember complex fractions?) $\frac{\frac{1}{2}}{49}$ is $\frac{1}{2} \div 49$.

$\frac{1}{2} \div \frac{49}{1} = \frac{1}{2} \times \frac{1}{49} = \frac{1}{98}$ (or 1 : 98)

$\frac{1}{2}$: 49 is the same as 1 : 98.

$\frac{1}{2}$ pound costs 49¢ and 1 pound costs 98¢.

Assume that 2 pounds of cake results from $3\frac{3}{4}$ cups of flour.

The ratio is $2 : 3\frac{3}{4}$ or $\frac{2}{3\frac{3}{4}}$.

$2 \div 3\frac{3}{4} = \frac{2}{1} \div \frac{15}{4} = \frac{2}{1} \times \frac{4}{15} = \frac{8}{15}$ (or 8 : 15)

So 2 pounds from $3\frac{3}{4}$ cups is the same as 8 pounds from 15 cups.

$2 : 3\frac{3}{4} = 8 : 15$.

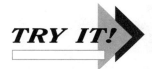

PRACTICE

Express each ratio as a common fraction. Reduce the fraction to lowest terms and state the ratio in lowest terms.

EXAMPLE

| 5 : 15 | $\frac{5}{15}$ | $\frac{1}{3}$ | 1 : 3 |

(The terms of the ratio 5 : 15 become the terms of the fraction $\frac{5}{15}$. Divide the numerator and denominator each by 5 to reduce. $\frac{5}{15} = \frac{1}{3}$. The terms of the fraction $\frac{1}{3}$ become the terms of the ratio 1 : 3.)

	RATIO	FRACTION	FRACTION	RATIO
1.	18 : 12	_____	_____	_____
2.	9 : 12	_____	_____	_____
3.	14 : 21	_____	_____	_____

Compare the following quantities using the correct ratio. Pay attention to the number labels. Write the answer in the lowest terms ratio.

In one class, 18 students are studying biology; 6 of the students are males.

4. female students compared to male students _____

5. male students compared to total students _____

6. female students compared to total students _____

7. male students compared to female students _____

(If there are 18 total students and 6 are males, then 12 are females).

ANSWERS

1. $\frac{18}{12} = \frac{3}{2} = 3:2$

2. $\frac{9}{12} = \frac{3}{4} = 3:4$

3. $\frac{14}{21} = \frac{2}{3} = 2:3$

4. females : males = 12 : 6 $\quad \frac{12}{6} = \frac{2}{1} \quad 2:1$

5. males : total = 6 : 18 $\quad \frac{6}{18} = \frac{1}{3} \quad 1:3$

6. females : total = 12 : 18 $\quad \frac{12}{18} = \frac{2}{3} \quad 2:3$

7. males : females = 6 : 12 $\quad \frac{6}{12} = \frac{1}{2} \quad 1:2$

Solution Strength as a Ratio

Ratios may be used to express the strength of a solution. Remember that a solution strength can also be stated in percent.

A. 1 : 25 solution

   1 part of pure drug is contained in 25 parts of solution ($1:25 = \frac{1}{25}$)

B. 1 : 40 solution

   1 part of pure drug is contained in 40 parts of solution ($1:40 = \frac{1}{40}$)

C. 1 : 1000 solution

   1 mL of pure liquid solute is contained in 1000 mL of solution ($1:1000 = 1\ mL/1000\ mL$)

   1 g of pure dry solute is contained in 1000 mL of solution ($1:1000 = 1\ g/1000\ mL$)

D. 1 : 20 solution

   1 g (or 1 mL) of pure drug is contained in 20 mL of solution ($1:20 = 1\ g/20\ mL$)

   $\frac{1}{20}$ is equivalent to $\frac{5}{100}$

   5 g (or 5 mL) of pure drug is contained in 100 mL of solution

   $\frac{5}{100}$ is equivalent to 5%

   A 1 : 20 solution is a 5% solution ($\frac{1}{20} = \frac{5}{100} = 5\%$)

Solution strength stated as a ratio means:
  grams of pure drug (dry) contained in milliliters of solution
  (grams : milliliters)

                              OR

milliliters of pure drug (liquid) contained in milliliters of solution
(milliliters: milliliters)

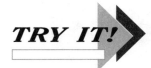

PRACTICE

1. A 1 : 50 solution is _____ part of pure drug contained in _____ parts of solution.
2. A 1 : 50 solution is 1 _____ or 1 _____ contained in 50 milliliters of solution.

ADDITIONAL PRACTICE

Fill in the chart. Do not reduce the ratio or fraction to lowest terms.

	RATIO	FRACTION	DECIMAL	PERCENT
3.	_____	$\frac{3}{5}$	_____	_____
4.	7 : 1	_____	_____	_____
5.	15 : 5	_____	_____	_____
6.	_____	$\frac{4}{20}$	_____	_____
7.	1 : 1	_____	_____	_____
8.	1 : 8	_____	_____	_____
9.	_____	$\frac{1}{10}$	_____	_____
10.	_____	$\frac{7}{8}$	_____	_____
11.	3 : 4	_____	_____	_____
12.	6 : 12	_____	_____	_____

Express each of the following as a ratio and its equivalent fraction. Use whole numbers for the terms of the ratio.

	RATIO	FRACTION
13. 3 g per capsule	_____	_____
14. 150 mg in (per) 3 tablets	_____	_____
15. 10 mg per tablet	_____	_____
16. 5 mg in (per) 10 mL	_____	_____
17. 2 g in 25 mL	_____	_____
18. $\frac{1}{2}$ lb for 30 cents	_____	_____
19. 20 miles per $\frac{1}{2}$ hour	_____	_____
20. 5 mL in 20 mL	_____	_____

Reduce each ratio to lowest terms.

21. 25 : 75 _____

22. 36 : 18 _____

ON THE JOB

Dosage strength is the weight of a drug contained in one tablet or capsule. For a liquid medication, dosage strength is the weight of a drug contained in a certain volume. Express each of the following as a lowest terms ratio and its equivalent fraction.

1. 20 mg per capsule _____ _____

2. 150 mg in 5 mL _____ _____

3. 5 grains per tablet _____ _____

4. 10 mg per milliliter _____ _____

5. 300 Units in 2 mL _____ _____

PART 4: PROPORTION

OBJECTIVES

1. *Understand the meaning of proportion.*
2. *Identify the mean and extreme terms in a proportion.*
3. *Prove the equality of a proportion using the means and extremes or cross multiplication.*

A proportion represents a relationship of equality between two ratios. There are four terms in a proportion; two terms from each ratio. The correct order of the four terms is critical to the understanding of the equality.

The Meaning of Proportion

A proportion is a statement that says two ratios are equal. Think also of a pair of equivalent fractions. A proportion can be expressed in two ways:

$$1 : 2 = 2 : 4 \quad \text{OR} \quad \frac{1}{2} = \frac{2}{4}$$

The = symbol in a proportion is read "as."

PROPORTION	EXPRESSED IN WORDS		
$1 : 2 = 2 : 4$	1 is to 2	as	2 is to 4
$\frac{9}{12} = \frac{3}{4}$	9 is to 12	as	3 is to 4
$2 : 6 = 3 : 9$	2 is to 6	as	3 is to 9
$\frac{3}{5} = \frac{6}{10}$	3 is to 5	as	6 is to 10

Observe very carefully the labels on the numbers in each ratio of the proportion.

A. If 3 apples cost 30 cents, then 6 apples cost 60 cents.
RATIO 3 apples for (compared to) 30 cents   3 apples : 30 cents
RATIO 6 apples for (compared to) 60 cents   6 apples : 60 cents

PROPORTION 3 apples : 30 cents = 6 apples : 60 cents
3 apples is to 30 cents as 6 apples is to 60 cents
3 : 30 = 6 : 60

The proportion states that the two ratios are equal. The ratio 3 : 30 in lowest terms is 1 : 10. The ratio 6 : 60 in lowest terms is 1 : 10.

The first terms of each ratio are related in some way. The second terms of each ratio correspond in some way as well. The 3 and 6 are related because they are both apples. The 30 and 60 are related because they are the *corresponding* costs of the apples.

B. If a distance of 45 miles can be traveled in 1 hour, then 90 miles can be traveled in 2 hours.

RATIO   45 miles per (compared to) 1 hour   45 miles : 1 hour

RATIO   90 miles per (compared to) 2 hours   90 miles : 2 hours

PROPORTION   45 miles : 1 hour = 90 miles : 2 hours
              45 miles is to 1 hour as 90 miles is to 2 hours
              45 : 1 = 90 : 2

The proportion is set up as miles : hours = miles : hours. The order of the labels is the same in each ratio.

The Means and the Extremes

Remember that a proportion states that two ratios are equal. The middle terms in a proportion are called the "means." The outer end terms are called the "extremes." The product of the means equals the product of the extremes.

A.

means

2 : 4 = 6 : 12

extremes

4 x 6   =   2 x 12
24   =   24

B. Think back to equivalent fractions that were verified by cross multiplication. Write the proportion 2 : 4 = 6 : 12 in fractional form. The product (multiplication answer) of one denominator times the opposite numerator equals the product of the other denominator times the opposite numerator.

24   24

$$\frac{2}{4} = \frac{6}{12}$$

C. To prove the equality of any proportion, the product of the means must equal the product of the extremes. This is the same cross product or cross multiplication rule that was used with equivalent fractions.

7 : 8 = 14 : 16   7 x 16 = 8 x 14
                              112   =   112
                              7 : 8 is equal to 14 : 16

3 : 4 ≠ 6 : 9   4 x 6 ≠ 3 x 9
                              24   ≠   27
                              3 : 4 is not equal to 6 : 9

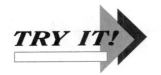

TRY IT!

PRACTICE

Express each true statement as a proportion.

1. If 20 milligrams are contained in 5 milliliters, then 80 milligrams are contained in 20 milliliters. _____

2. If 35 milligrams are contained in 1 capsule, then 70 milligrams are contained in 2 capsules. _____

3. If 10 mm equal a centimeter, then 78 mm equal 7.8 cm. _____

Test the equality of the proportions. (The product of the means equals the product of the extremes.) If the statement is true, fill in the symbol for equal (=). If the statement is not true, fill in the symbol for not equal (≠).

4. $9 : 15$ _____ $3 : 4$

5. $5 : 6$ _____ $30 : 36$

ANSWERS

1. $20 : 5$ = $80 : 20$
2. $35 : 1$ = $70 : 2$
3. $10 : 1$ = $78 : 7.8$
4. ≠
5. =

ADDITIONAL PRACTICE

Test the equivalence of the following proportions. Fill in the symbol (=) if the statement is true. Fill in the symbol (≠) if the statement is not true.

6. $75 : 100$ _____ $3 : 4$ 7. $6 : 9$ _____ $3 : 4\frac{1}{2}$

8. $5 : 8$ _____ $25 : 45$ 9. $\frac{1}{3} : \frac{2}{3}$ _____ $1 : 2$

10. $\frac{1}{4} : \frac{3}{4}$ _____ $1 : 4$ 11. $4 : 9$ _____ $80 : 180$

12. $75 : 125$ _____ $21 : 35$ 13. $12 : 3$ _____ $1 : 4$

14. $10 : 100$ _____ $2 : 20$ 15. $1 : 5$ _____ $4 : 4$

16. $\frac{2}{9}$ $\frac{6}{10}$ 17. $\frac{9}{21}$ $\frac{18}{42}$

18. $\frac{5}{4}$ $\frac{60}{48}$ 19. $\frac{8}{9}$ $\frac{34}{36}$

20. $\frac{8}{12}$ $\frac{24}{36}$

Express each true statement as a proportion.

1. If 50 mg are contained in 2 tablets, then 25 mg are contained in 1 tablet. _____

2. If 1 g is contained in 50 mL, then 5 g are contained in 250 mL. _____

3. If 1000 g equal a kilogram, then 2500 g equal 2.5 kilograms. _____

4. If 1 mL equals 1 cc, then 50 mL equal 50 cc. _____

5. If 1000 cc equal 1 L, then 4000 cc equal 4 L. _____

◆◆◆◆◆◆ **FUN FACTS** ◆◆◆◆◆◆

Blood type is an inherited trait and remains the same throughout life; 41% of the population have Type A blood; 45% have Type O blood; 10% have Type B blood; 4% have Type AB blood.

PART 5: COMPUTATIONS WITH PROPORTIONS

OBJECTIVES
1. *Solve for an unknown term in a proportion.*
2. *Convert measurement units using proportions.*

The ability to solve for an unknown quantity in a proportion is the basis of conversions between systems of measurement and dosage calculations. An accurate solution depends upon the correct placement of the four terms in the proportion.

Solving for an Unknown Term

Finding the missing term in a proportion is accomplished using cross multiplication or "the product of the means equals the product of the extremes."

In the following examples, note that multiplication is not represented with a times symbol (x). That could be confused with the unknown quantity, which is often shown as X.

A. $12 : X = 3 : 1$ Find the unknown term, X.

1. Write an equation.

Product of the means	=	Product of the extremes
Three times X	=	Twelve times one
3 X	=	12 (1)

2. To solve for the unknown, X must be isolated on one side of the equation. Divide each side of the equation by 3. (Doing exactly the same thing to each side keeps the equation balanced.)

$$3 X = 12$$

$$\frac{3 X}{3} = \frac{12}{3} \quad \left(\text{Note: } \frac{3}{3} = 1 \text{ and } 1 \text{ X} = \text{X}\right)$$

$$X = 4$$

3. Prove the equality of the proportion.

12 : 4	=	3 : 1
4 (3)	=	12 (1)
12	=	12

B. $25 : X = 4 : 5$ Find the missing term, X.

1. Write an equation.

Product of the means	=	Product of the extremes
Four times X	=	Five times twenty-five
4X	=	5 (25)
4X	=	125

2. Isolate the unknown and keep the equation balanced. Do exactly the same thing to each side of the equation. Divide by 4.

$$\frac{4\,X}{4} = \frac{125}{4} \quad \text{Note: } \frac{4}{4} = 1 \text{ and } 1\,X = X$$

$$X = 31.25$$

3. Prove the equality of the proportion.

$$25 : 31.25 = 4 : 5$$
$$4\,(31.25) = 5\,(25)$$
$$125 = 125$$

C. $\dfrac{X}{8} = \dfrac{18}{72}$

1. Write an equation based on the cross multiplication rule.

$$72\,X = 8\,(18)$$
$$72\,X = 144$$

2. Isolate the unknown, keeping the equation balanced.

$$\frac{72\,X}{72} = \frac{144}{72} \quad \text{Note: } \frac{72}{72} = 1 \text{ and } 1\,X = X$$

$$X = 2$$

3. Prove the equality of the proportion.

$$\frac{2}{8} = \frac{18}{72}$$

$$2\,(72) = 8\,(18)$$
$$144 = 144$$

D. 25 mg = _____ g. Use a proportion to convert 25 mg to grams. If 1000 mg = 1 g, then 25 mg = _____ g (1000 : 1 = 25 : X).

1. The first ratio should be the known equivalent between milligrams and grams (1000 mg = 1 g).

$$\frac{1000 \text{ mg}}{1 \text{ g}}$$

2. The second ratio must be set up so that the *same* labels are in exactly the *same* order as the first ratio (mg : g).

$$\frac{25 \text{ mg}}{X \text{ g}}$$

3. The two ratios are written in a proportion. (The labels are critical to proper conversion.)

EQUIVALENT		CONVERSION			
$\dfrac{1000 \text{ mg}}{1 \text{ g}}$	=	$\dfrac{25 \text{ mg}}{X \text{ g}}$	$\dfrac{1000}{1}$	=	$\dfrac{25}{X}$

4. Use cross multiplication to write an equation. Solve for the unknown quantity, X.

$$1000 \, X \quad = \quad 25$$

$$\frac{1000 \, X}{1000} \quad = \quad \frac{25}{1000}$$

$$X \quad = \quad 25/1000 \quad = \quad 0.025$$

5. $\dfrac{1000 \text{ mg}}{1 \text{ g}} \quad = \quad \dfrac{25 \text{ mg}}{0.025 \text{ g}}$

$25 \text{ mg} \quad = \quad 0.025 \text{ g}$

E. 0.75 L = _____ mL. Use a proportion to convert 0.75 L to milliliters. If 1000 mL = 1 L, then _____ mL = 0.75 L.

1. The first ratio should be the known equivalent between liters and milliliters (1000 mL = 1 L).

$$\frac{1000 \text{ mL}}{1 \text{ L}}$$

2. The second ratio contains the known quantity and the unknown quantity *in exactly the same label order* as the first ratio. (mL : L)

$$\frac{X \text{ mL}}{0.75 \text{ L}}$$

3. Set up a proportion. Use cross multiplication to write an equation and solve for X.

EQUIVALENT		CONVERSION			
$\dfrac{1000 \text{ mL}}{1 \text{ L}}$	=	$\dfrac{X \text{ mL}}{0.75 \text{ L}}$	$\dfrac{1000}{1}$	=	$\dfrac{X}{0.75}$

$1 \, X \quad = \quad 1000 \, (0.75)$
$X \quad = \quad 750$

4. $\dfrac{1000 \text{ mL}}{1 \text{ L}} \quad = \quad \dfrac{750 \text{ mL}}{0.75 \text{ L}}$

$0.75 \text{ L} \quad = \quad 750 \text{ mL}$

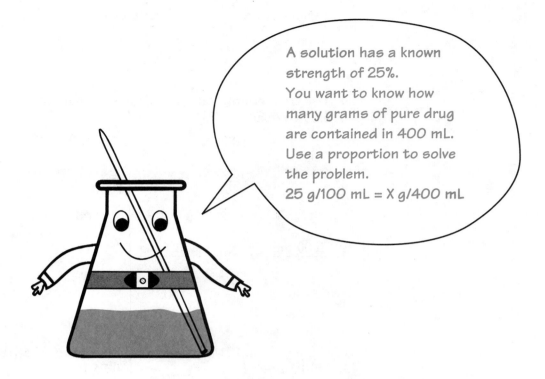

A solution has a known strength of 25%.
You want to know how many grams of pure drug are contained in 400 mL. Use a proportion to solve the problem.
25 g/100 mL = X g/400 mL

F. If a solution has a known strength of 25%, how many grams of pure drug are contained in 400 mL? Use a proportion to solve the problem.

1. The first ratio contains the *known information* about the solution strength. A 25% solution means 25 g of pure drug in 100 mL of solution (25 g / 100 mL).

$$\frac{25 \text{ g}}{100 \text{ mL}} = \underline{\hspace{2cm}}$$

2. The second ratio contains a known quantity and an unknown quantity in the *same label order* as the first ratio (g : mL).

$$\frac{X \text{ g}}{400 \text{ mL}}$$

3. The two ratios are written as a proportion.

$$\frac{25 \text{ g}}{100 \text{ mL}} = \frac{X \text{ g}}{400 \text{ mL}} \qquad \frac{25}{100} = \frac{X}{400}$$

4. Use cross multiplication to write an equation. Solve for the unknown quantity.

$$100 \text{ X} = 25 \, (400)$$

$$\frac{100 \text{ X}}{100} = \frac{10,000}{100}$$

$$\text{X} = 100$$

5. $$\frac{25 \text{ g}}{100 \text{ mL}} = \frac{100 \text{ g}}{400 \text{ mL}}$$

If 25 g of pure drug are contained in 100 mL, then 100 g of pure drug are contained in 400 mL of solution.

G. If a tablet contains 75 mg of medication, how many tablets contain 225 mg? Use a proportion to solve the problem.

1. Use the known information first.
   75 mg per tablet means 75 mg : 1 tablet. The ratio has an implied term of 1.

$$\frac{75 \text{ mg}}{1 \text{ tablet}}$$

2. Set up the second ratio in the same order as the first ratio (mg : tablet).

$$\frac{225 \text{ mg}}{\text{X tablets}}$$

3. Write the ratios as a proportion and solve for the unknown quantity.

$$\frac{75 \text{ mg}}{1 \text{ tablet}} = \frac{225 \text{ mg}}{\text{X tablet}} \qquad \frac{75}{1} = \frac{225}{\text{X}}$$

$$75 \text{ X} = 225$$

$$\frac{75 \text{ X}}{75} = \frac{225}{75}$$

$$\text{X} = 3$$

4. $$\frac{75 \text{ mg}}{1 \text{ tablet}} = \frac{225 \text{ mg}}{3 \text{ tablets}}$$

If 1 tablet contains 75 mg, then 3 tablets contain 225 mg.

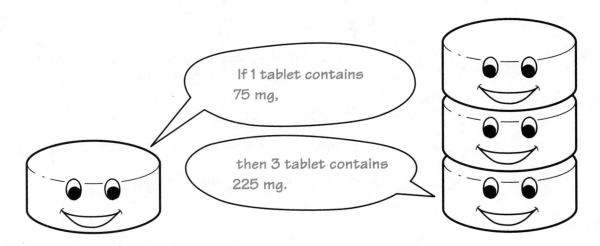

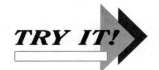

PRACTICE

Find the unknown quantity in each proportion. Use cross multiplication or "the product of the means equals the product of the extremes."

1. X : 15   =   1 : 3
2. 20 : 32   =   X : 48
3. $\dfrac{25}{70}$ = $\dfrac{X}{14}$

ANSWERS

1. X = 5
2. X = 30
3. X = 5

ADDITIONAL PRACTICE

Find the unknown quantity in each proportion. Express all answers in decimal form.

4. 1000 : 1   =   150 : X   X   =   _____

5. X : 100   =   5 : 20   X   =   _____

6. 8 : X   =   32 : 400   X   =   _____

7. 1 : 10   =   X : 75   X   =   _____

8. $\dfrac{1}{1000}$ = $\dfrac{X}{50}$ X   =   _____

9. $\dfrac{X}{3}$ = $\dfrac{25}{75}$ X   =   _____

10. $\dfrac{100}{5}$ = $\dfrac{X}{4}$ X   =   _____

11. $\dfrac{X}{2}$ = $\dfrac{15}{1.25}$ X   =   _____

12. $\dfrac{1}{1}$ = $\dfrac{95}{X}$ X   =   _____

13. $\dfrac{1}{2.2}$ = $\dfrac{X}{121}$ X   =   _____

Convert the following measurements using a proportion. Remember to use the known equivalent as the first ratio.

14. 750 mg   =   _____ g   15. 1.5 cc   =   _____ mL

16. 95 mm   =   _____ cm   17. 2050 g   =   _____ kg

18. 0.7 g   =   _____ mg

1. A terfenadine tablet contains 60 mg of medication. How many tablets contain 240 mg? _____

2. An ulcer medication has 300 mg in 2 tablets. How many milligrams are in 3 tablets? _____

3. A liquid medication contains 10 g in 100 mL. How many grams are contained in 5 mL? _____

4. A solution has a given strength of 20%. How many grams are in 50 mL of solution? _____

5. A 5% solution is in stock. How many milliliters contain 6 g? _____

◆◆◆◆◆◆ FUN FACTS ◆◆◆◆◆◆◆

The human brain is about 80% water.

EXERCISES

Express each fraction, decimal, and ratio as an equivalent percent.

1. $\frac{3}{2}$ = _____   2. 1 : 5 = _____

3. $\frac{7}{7}$ = _____   4. 20 to 100 = _____

5. 5 : 50 = _____   6. 1.5 = _____

7. $\frac{150}{600}$ = _____   8. $\frac{3}{5}$ = _____

9. 3 : 3 = _____   10. $\frac{1}{100}$ = _____

11. 0.75 = _____   12. 0.005 = _____

13. $\frac{1}{2}$ to 100 = _____   14. $\frac{1}{10}$ = _____

15. 1 to 1000 = _____   16. 0.5 = _____

17. 1 : 40 = _____   18. 1 = _____

19. 0.995 = _____   20. $\frac{1}{4}$ = _____

21. $\frac{3}{4}$ = _____   22. 150 : 50 = _____

23. 2 = _____   24. $\frac{1}{2}$ = _____

25. 17 to 17 = _____

Express each percent as a decimal.

26. 1% = _____   27. 10% = _____

28. 45% = _____   29. 3.5% = _____

30. 126% = _____   31. 75% = _____

32. 50% = _____   33. $6\frac{1}{2}$ % = _____

34. $4\frac{3}{4}$ % = _____   35. 25% = _____

36. 500% = _____   37. 100% = _____

38. 20% = _____   39. 98.2% = _____

40. $\frac{1}{2}$ % = _____

Express each of the following as a lowest terms ratio using whole numbers.

41. $\dfrac{\frac{1}{4}}{10}$ = _____ **42.** $\dfrac{18}{27}$ = _____

43. $\dfrac{9}{3}$ = _____ **44.** $\dfrac{100}{50}$ = _____

45. $\dfrac{5}{\frac{3}{4}}$ = _____ **46.** $1\frac{3}{4}$ = _____

47. $2\frac{5}{6}$ = _____ **48.** $\dfrac{25}{100}$ = _____

49. $\dfrac{\frac{1}{3}}{\frac{1}{2}}$ = _____ **50.** $\dfrac{30}{500}$ = _____

Determine if each of the following represents an equality or inequality. Use the product of the means equals the product of the extremes. Indicate the answer by inserting the = symbol or ≠ symbol.

51. 95 : 100 _____ 9 : 10 **52.** 1 : 10 _____ 2 : 100

53. $\frac{1}{2}$: 3 _____ 1 : 6 **54.** $\frac{1}{2}$: $\frac{2}{3}$ _____ 1 : $1\frac{1}{3}$

55. 0.5 : 4 _____ 1 : 7 **56.** 3 : 4 _____ 75 : 100

57. 1 : 20 _____ 5 : 100 **58.** 21 : 27 _____ 35 : 45

59. 1 : 3 _____ 7 : 8 **60.** 12 : 14 _____ 24 : 28

Write a lowest terms ratio to represent the indicated rate.

61. 100 mg in 4 tablets = _____

62. 20 mg contained in 10 mL = _____

63. 250 mcg per tablet = _____

64. 150 mg per 10 mL = _____

65. 500 mg in 4 tablets = _____

66. 1000 g in 1 kg = _____

67. 2 mL per 2 cc = _____

68. 100 cm in 1 m = _____

69. 1 meter contains 1000 mm   =   _____

70. 1000 mcg equal 1 mg   =   _____

71. 5 g per mL   =   _____

72. 90 mg contained in 9 mL   =   _____

73. 30 grains in 6 tablets   =   _____

74. 20 g contained in 20 mL   =   _____

75. 5 mg per 2 cc   =   _____

Find the unknown in each proportion. Express the answer in decimal form.

76. X : 12   =   18 : 24   X   =   _____

77. 7 : X   =   56 : 96   X   =   _____

78. 1 : 1000   =   X : 200   X   =   _____

79. 100 : 1   =   140 : X   X   =   _____

80. 3 : 4   =   75 : X   X   =   _____

81. 12 : 9   =   X : 27   X   =   _____

82. 1 : X   =   75 : 150   X   =   _____

83. X : 100   =   1 : 10   X   =   _____

84. 2.2 : 1   =   187 : X   X   =   _____

85. 1 : 1000   =   X : 50   X   =   _____

Find the unknown component in each proportion. Express answers in fractional form, if necessary.

86. $\dfrac{2}{3}$ = $\dfrac{X}{48}$ X = _____   **87.** $\dfrac{X}{\frac{1}{2}}$ = $\dfrac{14}{2}$ X = _____

88. $\dfrac{\frac{1}{2}}{\frac{5}{8}}$ = $\dfrac{4}{X}$ X = _____   **89.** $\dfrac{20}{100}$ = $\dfrac{X}{1000}$ X = _____

90. $\dfrac{X}{5}$ = $\dfrac{3}{20}$ X = _____

Convert the following measurements using proportions. Use the known equivalent as the first ratio.

91. _____ g   =   275 mg   **92.** _____ cm   =   1.75 m

93. 250 mcg   =   _____ mg   **94.** _____ m   =   50 cm

95. _____ mg   =   0.5 g   **96.** 205 g   =   _____ kg

97. 7.5 L   =   _____ mL   **98.** 0.5 mL   =   _____ cc

99. 0.25 g   =   _____ mg   **100.** 7 kg   =   _____ g

ON THE JOB

• • • • • • • • • •

1. Solution strength expressed as a percent means the number of _____ of dry solute in _____ mL of solution. Percent strength also means the number of _____ of liquid solute contained in 100 mL of solution.

Several stock solutions were in the supply cabinet. Solution strengths were expressed in percents or ratios. Indicate the amount of pure solute that is dissolved in the solution.

2. 1 : 25 solution   _____ g in _____ mL of solution

3. 5% solution   _____ g in _____ mL of solution

4. 3 : 10 solution   _____ mL in _____ mL of solution

5. 50% solution   _____ mL in _____ mL of solution

The following information is necessary for different dosage calculations. Convert each comparison to a ratio. (A ratio that compares quantities with unlike measurements is called a rate.)

6. 275 mg per tablet   =   _____

7. 50 mcg contained in a tablet   =   _____

8. 15 mg contained in 2 mL   =   _____

9. 1000 mg in a gram   =   _____

10. 1 kg equals 2.2 lb   =   _____

11. 0.5 g per capsule   =   _____

12. 1 mg equals 1000 mcg   =   _____

13. 1 T equals 3 tsp   =   _____

14. 4 mL equals 1 dram   =   _____

15. 1 mL is 1 cc   =   _____
Write each statement as a proportion.

16. There are 20 mcg of Drug A in a tablet so there are 80 mcg of Drug A in 4 tablets. _____

17. If there are 250 mg of Drug B in 15 mL, then there are 500 mg of Drug B in 30 mL. _____

18. If 1000 Units of Drug C are contained in 2 cc, then 500 Units of Drug C are contained in 1 cc. _____

19. There are 15 grains of medication in 3 tablets, so there are 5 grains in 1 tablet. _____

20. If 2.2 lb equals 1 kg, then 187 pounds equals 85 kg. _____

21. If 1000 mcg equals 1 mg, then 25 mcg equals 0.025 mg. _____

22. If a gram is equal to 1000 mg, then 0.4 g is equal to 400 mg. _____

23. A meter is equal to 100 cm. Therefore 0.75 m is equal to 75.0 cm. _____

24. If 5 mg are contained in 2 cc, then 2.5 mg are contained in 1 cc. _____

25. If 75 mg of Drug X are contained in 2 cc, then 112.5 mg of Drug X are contained in 3 cc. _____

26. If 70 mg are contained in 20 mL, then 210 mg are contained in 60 mL. _____

27. If 1 tablet contains 5 grains, then 4 tablets contain 20 grains. _____

28. If 75 mg are contained in 3 capsules, then 50 mg are contained in 2 capsules. _____

29. If 1000 mg equal a gram, then 500 mg equal 0.5 g. _____

30. If 1 kg equals 2.2 lb, then 14 kg equals 30.8 lb. _____

Set up a proportion and solve for the missing component.

31. A capsule contains 325 mg. How many capsules contain 1300 mg? _____

32. 400 mg of Drug Z are contained in 5 mL. How many milliliters contain 200 mg? _____

33. How many milligrams are equal to 0.8 g? _____

34. 10 mg of Drug Y are delivered in 1 milliliter. How many milligrams are in 3 cc? _____

35. How many grams are equal to 750 mg? _____

36. How many micrograms are equal to 0.4 mg? _____

37. A milliliter contains 0.4 mg of Drug T. How many milligrams are in 3 cc (3 mL)? _____

38. How many centimeters are equal to 1.75 m? _____

39. 10 mg of Drug R are contained in 2 cc. How many cubic centimeters (cc) contain 3 mg? _____

40. 100 mg of Drug M are contained in 2 cc. How many cubic centimeters (cc) contain 5 mg? _____

◆◆◆◆◆◆ **FUN FACTS** ◆◆◆◆◆◆

About 21 pounds of milk is needed to make one pound of butter (21 : 1).

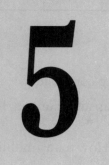

UNIT 5

Systems of Weight and Measure

OBJECTIVES

1. *Identify the common units of volume and weight in the apothecaries' system of measurement.*
2. *List the volume equivalents within the apothecaries' system.*

The apothecaries' system is a very old English system of measurement. (An apothecary is a person who prepares and dispenses drugs; that is, a druggist or pharmacist.) Although it is being replaced by the metric system, some units of the apothecaries' system are still in use today. Therefore, it is important to understand both systems.

Weight

In the apothecaries' system, the grain (gr) is the basic unit of weight. When the system was established, the weight of a grain of wheat was chosen as the basic unit. A grain is approximately the weight of a drop of water. There are, of course, larger units of weight, but the grain (gr) is the most common of the apothecaries' weight units in use today in the field of medicine. The symbols for grain (gr) and gram (g) are similar, but they do represent different quantities.

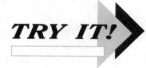

PRACTICE

1. The basic unit of weight in the apothecaries' system is the _____.

2. The symbol for grain is _____.

3. One grain is approximately the weight of a _____ of water.

ANSWERS

1. grain
2. gr
3. drop

Volume

The minim (m_x) is the basic unit of volume in the apothecaries' system. It can be thought of as nearly equal in volume to a drop. It was originally defined as the quantity of water that weighed the same as a grain of wheat. Basically, this very small unit has become obsolete as a unit of volume.

The apothecaries' units of volume used most often in drug measurement are the dram (℥) and the ounce (℥). Notice the scale on the medicine cup: 8 drams is equal to 1 ounce.

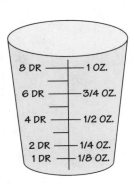

A dram is a smaller unit than an ounce. Think of the symbol for the dram as a "z" with a tail (℥). Think of the symbol for ounce as having a "greater than symbol" (>) on top of the "z" with a tail (℥).

Remember, the ounce is a larger unit of volume and the symbol for ounce is a larger symbol. A mistake in the understanding of the symbols could be very serious because of the difference in the measures.

Consider for a moment that a dram (℥) equals 4 mL. A dram or 4 mL of liquid will just cover the bottom of a medicine cup. An ounce, on the other hand, equals 30 mL, which is a full medicine cup.

Additional units of volume are pints (pt), quarts (qt), and gallons (gal); 16 ounces (℥) of liquid equal a pint, 2 pints equal a quart, and 4 quarts equal a gallon.

The volume equivalents within the apothecaries' system should be memorized.

APOTHECARIES' SYSTEM VOLUME EQUIVALENTS			
1 ounce	=	8 drams	
1 pint	=	16 ounces	
1 quart	=	2 pints	= 32 ounces
1 gallon	=	4 quarts	

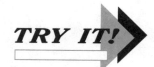

TRY IT!

PRACTICE

1. The basic unit of volume in the apothecaries' system is the _____.

2. The units of volume in the apothecaries' system that are most often used in drug measurements are the _____ and the _____.

3. The symbol for dram is _____.

4. The symbol for ounce is _____.

5. The dram is a (larger, smaller) unit than the ounce.

6. 1 ounce = _____ drams

7. 1 pint = _____ ounces

8. 1 quart = _____ pints

9. _____ quarts = 1 gallon

10. _____ ounce = 8 drams

ANSWERS

1. minim
2. dram, ounce
3. ʒ
4. ℥
5. smaller
6. 8
7. 16
8. 2
9. 4
10. 1

◆◆◆◆◆◆ **FUN FACTS** ◆◆◆◆◆◆

It takes a scant 1 1/2 ounces of wax to construct a honeycomb that would hold 4 pounds of honey.

PART 2: APOTHECARIES' SYSTEM: NOTATION AND SYMBOLS

OBJECTIVES

1. *Interpret apothecaries' measurements stated in symbolic notation.*
2. *Express apothecaries' measurements in proper symbolic notation.*
3. *List the volume equivalents within the apothecaries' system of measurement.*

It is necessary to understand the symbols and notation associated with the apothecaries' units that are still in use today. Symbolic notation in the apothecaries' system of measurement is the opposite of standard metric notation.

Symbolic Notation

Review the symbols that have already been introduced.

For weight:	grain	gr
For volume:	minim	♏
	dram	ʒ (dr)
	ounce	℥ (oz)
	pint	pt
	quart	qt
	gallon	gal

In the apothecaries' system, common fractions are used to express amounts less than one whole, except for the fraction $\frac{1}{2}$, which is represented by a special symbol (ss). The symbol (ss) comes from the Latin word semis which means one-half. (In the metric system decimals are always used; decimals are never used in the apothecaries' system.) Here are the common fractions used most often in the apothecaries' system:

$$\frac{1}{16} \qquad \frac{1}{8} \qquad \frac{1}{4} \qquad \text{ss} \qquad \frac{3}{4}$$

Whole numbers are most often expressed in lowercase Roman numerals, although Arabic numerals are used in certain circumstances. Apothecary amounts of 10 or less are written in lowercase Roman numerals; amounts greater than 10, except 20 (xx) and 30 (xxx), are written in Arabic numerals.

NUMBER	ROMAN NUMERAL (CAPITAL)	ROMAN NUMERAL (LOWERCASE)
one	I	i
two	II	ii
three	III	iii
four	IV	iv
five	V	v
six	VI	vi
seven	VII	vii
eight	VIII	viii
nine	IX	ix
ten	X	x
twenty	XX	xx
thirty	XXX	xxx

If the measurement unit is written out in full, Arabic numerals are used preceding the unit.

3 grains	$7\frac{1}{2}$ grains	$\frac{1}{4}$ grain
2 pints	5 drams	$\frac{3}{4}$ ounces
12 ounces	3 quarts	$2\frac{1}{2}$ ounces

If the *symbol* for the measurement unit is used, Roman numerals in lowercase are used following the symbol. Arabic numerals are often used if the quantity is greater than 10, but not 20 (xx) or 30 (xxx).

Remember, symbolic notation in the apothecaries' system is the opposite of metric notation. In the metric system, the quantity is stated first using decimals and the symbol is second. In the apothecaries' system, the symbol is first and the quantity is second using common fractions if necessary.

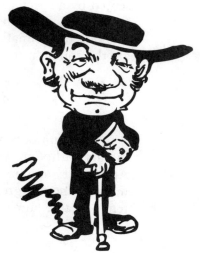

Words to live by: If the measurement unit is written out in full, Arabic numerals are used preceding the unit.

SYMBOLIC NOTATION	MEANING
gr ss	$\frac{1}{2}$ grain
gr iii	3 grains
gr viiss	$7\frac{1}{2}$ grains
gr $\frac{1}{4}$	$\frac{1}{4}$ grain
gr x	10 grains
gr xxx	30 grains
ʒ v	5 drams
ʒ iv	4 drams
ʒ iiss	$2\frac{1}{2}$ drams
℥ xx	20 ounces
℥ 12	12 ounces
℥ viii	8 ounces
pt ii	2 pints
qt	1 quart

Here's a summary of apothecaries' system volume equivalents and symbols for review.

SYMBOLIC NOTATION	MEANING
℥ i = ʒ viii	1 ounce = 8 drams
pt i = ℥ 16	1 pint = 16 ounces
qt i = pt ii	1 quart = 2 pints
gal i = qt iv	1 gallon = 4 quarts

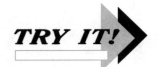

PRACTICE

Write the meaning of the symbol.

1. ℨ   _____   **2.** gr   _____

3. ss   _____   **4.** ♏   _____

5. ℥   _____

Write the correct apothecaries' notation using symbols.

6. $6 \frac{1}{2}$ drams   _____   **7.** 30 grains   _____

8. 16 ounces   _____   **9.** $\frac{1}{8}$ grain   _____

10. $2 \frac{1}{4}$ drams   _____

ANSWERS

1. dram	**2.** grain
3. $\frac{1}{2}$	**4.** minim
5. ounce	**6.** ℨ viss
7. gr xxx	**8.** ℥ 16
9. gr $\frac{1}{8}$	**10.** ℨ ii $\frac{1}{4}$

◆◆◆◆◆◆◆ FUN FACTS ◆◆◆◆◆◆◆

Twenty-seven thousand spider webs weigh about a pound.

ADDITIONAL PRACTICE

Write the meaning of the notations.

11. ℥ viss _____   **12.** gr ix   _____

13. ℈ xxx _____   **14.** gr $\frac{1}{6}$ _____

15. ℈ iiiss _____

Write the measurements in symbolic notation.

16. 4 $\frac{1}{2}$ ounces _____   **17.** 5 drams   _____

18. 20 drams _____   **19.** 8 $\frac{1}{4}$ grains   _____

20. 12 ounces _____

Fill in the blanks to form correct volume equivalents in symbols.

21. ℈ _____ = ℥ i   **22.** pt i   =   _____ 16

23. qt i   =   pt _____   **24.** gal i   =   qt _____

25. ℈ i   =   _____ viii

ON THE JOB

Read the physician's orders for the medications. Write the meaning of the dosage which is stated in apothecaries' notation.

1. Maalox   ℈ iv   _____

2. aspirin   gr 15   _____

3. aluminum phosphate   ℈ i   _____

The drug label on medicines states the dosage strength of the drug (the amount of the drug by weight). Write the meaning of the drug strength which is given in apothecaries' notation.

4. phenobarbital gr ss   tablet   _____

5. scopolamine hydrobromide
     gr $\frac{1}{300}$ tablet   _____

PART 3: CONVERSION WITHIN THE APOTHECARIES' SYSTEM

OBJECTIVES

1. *List the volume equivalents within the apothecaries' system of measurement.*
2. *Convert from one volume unit to another within the apothecaries' system.*

Conversion of weight units within the apothecaries' system is unnecessary because the emphasis here is placed only on one weight unit, the grain (gr). Conversion between units of volume within the system can be accomplished using conversion factors or proportions.

Volume Conversions

Here are some volume equivalents used in the apothecaries' system that you should know.

APOTHECARIES' SYSTEM VOLUME EQUIVALENTS				
℥	i	=	ʒ	viii
pt	i	=	℥	16
qt	i	=	pt	ii
gal	i	=	qt	iv

A. Express 20 drams as ounces.

1. Write a proportion using the known equivalent for the first ratio (8 drams to 1 ounce).

$$\frac{8 \text{ drams}}{1 \text{ ounce}} = \text{\underline{\hspace{3cm}}}$$

2. The second ratio contains the quantity that is given and the quantity to be found. It must follow the exact sequence of the first ratio. The labels in the numerators must match and the labels in the denominators must match.

$$\frac{8 \text{ drams}}{1 \text{ ounce}} = \frac{20 \text{ drams}}{X \text{ ounces}} \qquad \frac{8}{1} = \frac{20}{X}$$

3. Cross multiply.

$$8X = 20$$

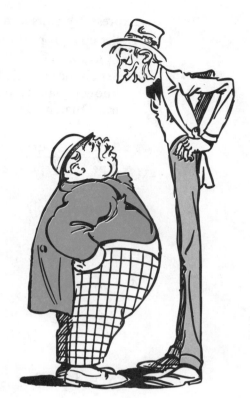

Drams is to ounces like short is to tall.

4. Solve for X.

$$\frac{8X}{8} = \frac{20}{8}$$

$$X = \frac{20}{8} = 2\frac{4}{8} = 2\frac{1}{2} \text{ ounces}$$

5. 20 drams = $2\frac{1}{2}$ ounces OR ℥ xx = ℥ iiss

B. Express 6 ounces as drams.
   1. Equivalent? 1 ounce = 8 drams (8 is the conversion factor)
   2. Multiply or Divide? The conversion is to smaller units. Multiply by the conversion factor, 8.

   6 x 8 = 48 drams

   3. 6 ounces = 48 drams OR ℥ vi = ℥ 48

C. Express $3\frac{1}{2}$ pints as quarts.
1. Set up a proportion using the known equivalent as the first ratio (1 qt to 2 pt).
2. Set up the second ratio in the same sequence as the first, using the known quantity and the quantity to be found. Numerator labels must match. Denominator labels must match.

$$\frac{1 \text{ qt}}{2 \text{ pt}} = \frac{X \text{ qt}}{3\frac{1}{2} \text{ pt}} \qquad \frac{1}{2} = \frac{X}{3\frac{1}{2}}$$

3. Cross multiply.

$$2X = 3\frac{1}{2}$$

4. Solve for X.

$$\frac{2X}{2} = \frac{3\frac{1}{2}}{2}$$

$$X = 3\frac{1}{2} \div 2 = \frac{7}{2} \div \frac{2}{1} = \frac{7}{2} \times \frac{1}{2} = \frac{7}{4} = 1\frac{3}{4} \text{ qt}$$

5. $3\frac{1}{2}$ pints $= 1\frac{3}{4}$ quarts OR pt iiiss = qt i $\frac{3}{4}$

D. Express 56 ounces as pints.
1. Equivalent? 1 pint = 16 ounces
2. Multiply or Divide? The conversion is to larger units. Divide by the conversion factor, 16.

$$\frac{56}{16} = 3\frac{1}{2} \text{ pints}$$

3. 56 ounces = $3\frac{1}{2}$ pints OR ℥ 56 = pt iiiss

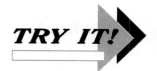

TRY IT!

PRACTICE

Convert from one apothecaries' volume unit to another using proportions or conversion factors. Express the equivalency in symbolic notation.

1. Express $3\frac{3}{4}$ ounces as drams. _____

2. Express 36 drams as ounces. _____

ANSWERS

1. ℥ iii $\frac{3}{4}$ = ℨ xxx

$$\frac{8 \text{ drams}}{1 \text{ ounce}} = \frac{X \text{ drams}}{3\frac{3}{4} \text{ ounces}}$$

$$X = 8\left(3\frac{3}{4}\right) = \left(\frac{8}{1}\right)\left(\frac{15}{4}\right) = \frac{120}{4} = 30 \text{ drams}$$

2. ℨ 36 = ℥ ivss

$$\frac{8 \text{ drams}}{1 \text{ ounce}} = \frac{36 \text{ drams}}{X \text{ ounces}}$$

$$8X = 36$$

$$\frac{8X}{8} = \frac{36}{8}$$

$$X = 4\frac{4}{8} = 4\frac{1}{2} \text{ ounces}$$

ADDITIONAL PRACTICE

Express the equivalents in symbolic notation.

3. ℥ _____ = ℨ ii

4. ℥ i $\frac{1}{4}$ = ℨ _____

5. ℥ 32 = pt _____

6. ℨ 24 = ℥ _____

7. ℨ _____ = ℥ ss

8. ℨ 12 = ℥ _____

9. ℥ _____ = ℨ vi

10. qt _____ = pt iii

11. ℨ xxx = ℥ _____

12. ℥ ii ss = ℨ _____

OBJECTIVES

1. *Identify the common units of volume in the household system of measurement.*
2. *List the volume equivalents within the household system.*
3. *Express household measurements in symbolic notation.*
4. *Convert from one volume unit to another within the household system.*

The household system is a much less accurate system of measurement than the apothecaries' or metric. This system is often used by a patient in a home setting, using common household utensils for measurement. It is not used in the hospital administration of drugs, but it may be necessary to explain take-home prescriptions to a patient in terms of familiar household units. All of the units explained here are units of volume (capacity).

Units of Volume

The basic unit in the household system is the drop (gtt), which varies in amount according to the diameter of the measuring utensil. Other units include the teaspoon (t or tsp), the tablespoon (T or tbs), the teacupful, and the glassful. The inaccuracy of the system is apparent in the units.

There is no formal system of symbolic notation in the household system. Quantities are generally expressed in Arabic numerals preceding an abbreviation, for example, 3 T, 2 tsp, 5 gtt.

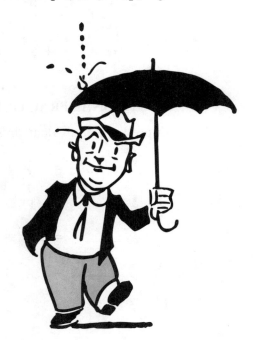

So the drop isn't accurate. Neither is the tablespoon which is equal to about 3 teaspoons.

<table>
<tr><th colspan="3">HOUSEHOLD SYSTEM
UNITS OF VOLUME</th></tr>
<tr><th>UNIT</th><th>ABBREVIATION</th><th>EQUIVALENT</th></tr>
<tr><td>drop</td><td>gtt</td><td></td></tr>
<tr><td>teaspoon</td><td>t (or tsp)</td><td></td></tr>
<tr><td>tablespoon</td><td>T (or tbs)</td><td>1 T = 3 tsp</td></tr>
<tr><td>teacup</td><td></td><td></td></tr>
<tr><td>glass</td><td></td><td></td></tr>
</table>

There is only one equivalent *within* the household system that is meaningful in drug measurement. It should be memorized.

$$1 \text{ T} = 3 \text{ t} \quad \text{or} \quad 1 \text{ tbs} = 3 \text{ tsp}$$

Note that the tablespoon (abbreviated with a capital letter) is a larger unit of measurement than the teaspoon (abbreviated with a lowercase letter). Conversion of units within the household system can be accomplished using proportions or conversion factors.

A. Express $2\frac{1}{3}$ tablespoons as teaspoons.

1. Write a proportion using the known equivalent as the first ratio (1 T to 3 tsp). Set up the second ratio with the quantity that is given and the quantity to be found. The same sequence of labels *must* be used for both ratios.

$$\frac{1 \text{ T}}{3 \text{ t}} = \frac{2\frac{1}{3} \text{ T}}{\text{X t}} \qquad \text{OR} \qquad \frac{1}{3} = \frac{2\frac{1}{3}}{\text{X}}$$

2. Cross multiply and solve for X.

$$\text{X} = 3(2\frac{1}{3})$$

$$\text{X} = \frac{3}{1}\left(\frac{7}{3}\right) = \frac{7}{1} = 7 \text{ t}$$

3. $2\frac{1}{3} \text{ T} = 7 \text{ t}$

B. Express 8 teaspoons as tablespoons.
   1. Equivalent? 1 T = 3 tsp. The conversion factor is 3.
   2. Multiply or Divide? The conversion is to larger units. Divide by the conversion factor.

$$\frac{8}{3} = 2\frac{2}{3}\ T$$

   3. 8 t = $2\frac{2}{3}$ T

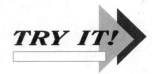

PRACTICE

1. The least accurate system of measurement is the (apothecaries', household, metric) system.

2. One tablespoon equals _____ teaspoons.

3. Fill in the abbreviations for the household units.

   drop   _____

   teaspoon   _____   or   _____

   tablespoon _____   or   _____

4. Calculate the equivalent measure.

   $4\frac{2}{3}$ T   =   _____ t

   15 t   =   _____ T

ADDITIONAL PRACTICE

Calculate the equivalent measures.

5. _____ t = $2\frac{1}{3}$ T   6. 1 t   = _____ T

7. 1 T   = _____ t   8. 2 t   = _____ T

9. _____ t = 3 T   10. _____ T = 4 t

11. _____ T = 23 t   12. 7 T   = _____ t

13. 12 t   = _____ T   14. _____ t = $4\frac{2}{3}$ T

PART 5: APOTHECARY/METRIC/HOUSEHOLD CONVERSION

OBJECTIVES

1. *List the weight and volume equivalents between the apothecaries', metric, and household systems of measurement.*
2. *Convert weight measurements between the apothecaries' and metric systems of measurement.*
3. *Convert volume measurements between the apothecaries', metric, and household systems of measurement.*

In addition to converting units within a system of measurement, it is important to be able to convert units between systems of measurement. An available or on-hand supply of a drug is not always measured in the same system in which a drug is prescribed.

Conversion between Systems of Measurement

Conversion of units between systems of measurement is most safely accomplished with proportions, using the known equivalent as the first ratio in the proportion. The second ratio is set up with the same sequence of labels as the first ratio. The given quantity and the quantity to be found are the terms of the second ratio.

The chart lists the most commonly used conversions (for drug measurement) between the apothecaries', metric, and household systems of measurement. **Conversion factors between systems of measurement are not exact, because the units from one system to another are not exact multiples of one another.** The conversions listed between systems are commonly accepted approximate equivalents that are within safe limits for drug administration. Memorize the weight and volume equivalents.

WEIGHT EQUIVALENTS

APOTHECARY		METRIC
1 grain (gr)	=	60 milligrams (mg)
15 grains (gr)	=	1 gram (g)

VOLUME EQUIVALENTS

APOTHECARY		METRIC		HOUSEHOLD
1 minim (m)	=			1 drop (gtt)
1 dram (ʒ)	=	4 mL (4 cc)		
		5 mL (5 cc)	=	1 teaspoon (t)
		15 mL (15 cc)	=	1 tablespoon (T)
1 ounce (ʒ)	=	30 mL (30 cc)	=	2 tablespoons (T)

A. Express 150 milligrams as grains.
   1. Write a proportion using the known equivalent as the first ratio (1 grain = 60 milligrams).

   $$\frac{1 \text{ grain}}{60 \text{ milligrams}} = \frac{X \text{ grains}}{150 \text{ milligrams}} \qquad \frac{1}{60} = \frac{X}{150}$$

   2. Use cross multiplication to solve for the unknown quantity.

   $$60 X = 150$$

   $$\frac{60 X}{60} = \frac{150}{60}$$

   $$X = 2\frac{1}{2} \text{ grains}$$

   3. 150 mg = gr iiss

B. Express 2.4 grams as grains.
   1. Write a proportion using the known equivalent as the first ratio (1 gram = 15 grains).

   $$\frac{15 \text{ grains}}{1 \text{ gram}} = \frac{X}{2.4 \text{ grams}} \qquad \frac{15}{1} = \frac{X}{2.4}$$

   2. Use cross multiplication to solve for X.

   $$X = 15(2.4)$$
   $$X = 36 \text{ grains}$$

   3. 2.4 g = gr 36

C. _____ mL = 4 teaspoons
   1. Set up an appropriate proportion using the known equivalent as the first ratio. Cross multiply and solve for the unknown quantity.

   $$\frac{5 \text{ mL}}{1 \text{ tsp}} = \frac{X \text{ mL}}{4 \text{ tsp}} \qquad \frac{5}{1} = \frac{X}{4}$$

   $$X = 20$$

   2. 20 mL = 4 tsp

D. 16 mL = _____ drams

    1. Set up an appropriate proportion using the known equivalent as the first ratio. Cross multiply and solve for the unknown quantity.

$$\frac{4\ mL}{1\ dram} = \frac{16\ mL}{X\ dram} \quad OR \quad \frac{4}{1} = \frac{16}{X}$$

$$4\ X = 16$$

$$\frac{4\ X}{4} = \frac{16}{4}$$

$$X = 4$$

    2. 16 mL = 4 drams

E. 75 mL = _____ ounces

    1. Set up an appropriate proportion using the known equivalent as the first ratio. Cross multiply and solve for the unknown quantity.

$$\frac{1\ oz}{30\ mL} = \frac{X\ oz}{75\ mL} \quad OR \quad \frac{1}{30} = \frac{X}{75}$$

$$30\ X = 75$$

$$\frac{30\ X}{30} = \frac{75}{30}$$

$$X = 2\frac{15}{30} = 2\frac{1}{2}$$

    2. 75 mL = $2\frac{1}{2}$ oz

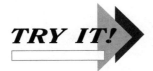

PRACTICE

Use proportions to convert the weight units between systems of measurement. Express the equivalent in correct symbolic notation. (Remember: 1 grain = 60 mg and 15 grains = 1 gram)

1. gr xss   = _____ g   **2.** 660 mg = gr _____

3. 0.6 g   = gr _____   **4.** gr vss = _____ mg

5. ℥ ss   = _____ mL   **6.** 20 mL = _____ t sp

ADDITIONAL PRACTICE

7. ℥ _____ = $4\frac{1}{2}$ T

8. 4 tsp = _____ mL

9. _____ mL = 5 tbs

10. ℈ vii = _____ mL

11. ℥ _____ = 45 mL

12. _____ T = 54 mL

13. 45 mL = _____ t

14. gr _____ = 210 mg

15. 22 mL = ℥ _____

16. _____ mg = gr ivss

17. _____ g = gr iii

18. ℥ vi = _____ tbs

19. gr _____ = 0.5 g

20. _____ mL = ℥ iv

21. gr v = _____ mg

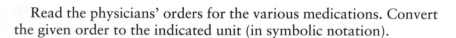

ON THE JOB

Read the physicians' orders for the various medications. Convert the given order to the indicated unit (in symbolic notation).

1. phenobarbital, 15 mg   gr _____

2. aminophylline, gr viiss   _____ g

3. pentobarbital, gr iss   _____ mg

4. Tylenol, 2 t   _____ mL

5. Gelusil ℥ i   _____ T

PART 6: OTHER DRUG MEASURES

OBJECTIVES

1. *Identify units (U) as drug dosage measurements.*
2. *Identify milliequivalents (mEq) as drug dosage measurements.*

Quantities of drugs may also be indicated in Units (U) or milliequivalents (mEq). Conversions for either milliequivalents or Units are unnecessary. Drugs in these measurements are prescribed, prepared, and administered all in the same system.

Units and Milliequivalents

A Unit (not a weight measurement) is an amount of a drug which produces a certain effect. The meaning of the Unit varies with the particular drug being measured, since the amounts and related effects of various drugs differ. Insulin is a familiar drug administered in Units.

A milliequivalent is a measurement of the weight of a drug contained in a certain volume of solution.

The quantity of Units or milliequivalents is expressed in Arabic numerals followed by the appropriate symbol, U or mEq.

Review these definitions.

SYMBOLIC NOTATION	MEANING
10,000 U	10,000 Units
20 mEq	20 milliequivalents

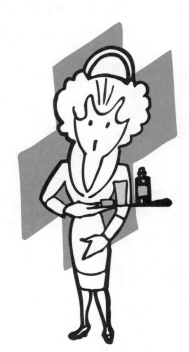

Remember: A Unit is an amount of a drug which produces a certain effect.

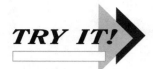
TRY IT!

PRACTICE

Interpret the notation. Write the meaning in the blank.

1. 1000 U _____

2. 2 mEq _____

ANSWERS

1. 1,000 Units
2. 2 milliequivalents

▲▲▲▲▲▲▲▲▲▲▲▲▲▲▲▲▲▲▲▲▲▲▲▲▲▲▲▲▲▲▲▲▲

◆◆◆◆◆◆◆ **FUN FACTS** ◆◆◆◆◆◆◆

The average American male child reaches half of his adult height at the age of two years.

EXERCISES

Identify the symbol or abbreviation.

1. U _____

2. gtt _____

3. g _____

4. ʒ _____

5. mEq _____

6. qt _____

7. ℥ _____

8. mg _____

9. tsp _____

10. m̨ _____

11. gr _____

12. mL _____

13. tbs _____

14. cc _____

15. t _____

16. pt _____

17. dr _____

18. T _____

19. gal _____

20. oz _____

Express each measurement in correct symbolic notation.

21. $5\frac{1}{2}$ grains _____

22. 5000 Units _____

23. $2\frac{3}{4}$ grams _____

24. 20 drams _____

25. 10 pints _____

26. 3 milliequivalents _____

27. $2\frac{3}{4}$ ounces _____

28. 4 teaspoons _____

29. 2 tablespoons _____

30. $\frac{1}{100}$ grain _____

Interpret the symbolic notation.

31. gr xxx _____

32. qt iv _____

33. ʒ vi _____

34. 100 U _____

35. ℥ ix _____

36. 4 gtt _____

37. gr $\frac{1}{20}$ _____

38. m̨ 15 _____

39. 2 T _____

40. 3 t _____

Express an equivalent measurement of volume.

41. 7 T = _____ t

42. ℨ _____ = 14 mL

43. 1.5 cc = _____ mL

44. _____ mL = ℥ ss

45. ℨ v = ℥ _____

46. _____ mL = 7 t

47. ℨ _____ = ℥ i $\frac{1}{4}$

48. 30 mL = _____ T

49. 2 mL = _____ cc

50. _____ t = 24 mL

51. _____ tbs = 12 tsp

52. _____ T = 15 mL

53. ℨ ii = _____ mL

54. _____ mL = 2.5 cc

55. 22.5 mL = ℥ _____

Express an equivalent weight.

56. 0.75 g = gr _____

57. gr ii $\frac{1}{4}$ = _____ mg

58. _____ g = 60 mg

59. gr vi = _____ g

60. 105 mg = gr _____

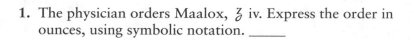

ON THE JOB

1. The physician orders Maalox, ℥ iv. Express the order in ounces, using symbolic notation. _____

Read the physician's order. Write the meaning of the dosage which is stated in notation.

2. caffeine   gr iii   _____

3. terpin hydrate   ℨ iii   _____

4. aspirin   gr x   _____

5. phenobarbital   gr $\frac{1}{4}$ _____

6. Tylenol   2 tsp   _____

7. The physician orders Kaopectate, ℥ ii. Express the order in drams, using symbolic notation. _____

Write the meaning of the drug strength which is stated on the drug label.

8. methyldopa gr viiss tablet _____

9. morphine sulfate gr $\frac{1}{4}$ tablet _____

10. aspirin gr v tablet _____

11. dimenhydrate gr $\frac{5}{6}$ tablet _____

12. sodium bicarbonate gr ivss tablet _____

13. The physician orders Benadryl, ℥ iii. Express the order in ounces, using symbolic notation. _____

14. An order is filled for $\frac{1}{2}$ quart of orange juice. Express the quantity in pints. _____

Convert the dosage strength which is given in grams or milligrams to grains.

15. digitoxin   0.1 mg   gr _____

16. phenobarbital   0.015 g   gr _____

17. amitriptyline hydrochloride   100 mg   gr _____

18. morphine sulfate   30 mg   gr _____

19. morphine sulfate   0.005 g   gr _____

20. The physician orders 3 tsp of cough medication. Express the order in tablespoons. _____

Convert the dosage strength in grains to milligrams or grams, as indicated.

21. atropine sulfate   gr $\frac{1}{200}$ _____ mg

22. calcium lactate   gr x   _____ mg

23. nadolol   gr ii   _____ mg

24. pentobarbital   gr iss   _____ g

25. caffeine   gr iii   _____ g

6

Dosage Calculations

OBJECTIVES

1. *Identify the basic equipment used in the administration of medication.*
2. *Identify various syringes by total volume, use, and calibration.*
3. *Read a given volume of medication contained in a syringe.*

Various types of vessels are used for the administration of medication. In order to become familiar with the uses and calibrations of common equipment, a brief overview is presented. (Remember that when dealing with volume and dosage calculations, 1 mL is equal to 1 cc.)

Oral Administration

The medicine cup is a small plastic container which is labeled in milliliters (mL), cubic centimeters (cc), drams (dr), ounces (oz), teaspoons (tsp), or tablespoons (tbs). It is used to administer liquid medication orally.

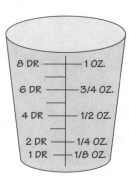
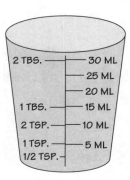

When administering an oral dosage of less than 5 mL or liquid medication to a child, an oral syringe is sometimes preferable to a medicine cup. Calibrated droppers are usually supplied with the specific medication for which they are intended. Calibrated droppers are not uniformly manufactured and the diameter of the dropper opening determines the size of the drops. For this reason, medications which come with droppers should be measured only in those droppers.

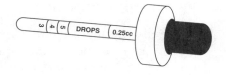

Parenteral Administration Syringes

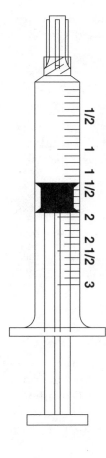

All syringes are measured in cubic centimeters (cc) or milliliters (mL) with the calibrations (individual markings) being in whole cc, tenths (0.1) of a cc, 2 tenths (0.2) of a cc, or hundredths (0.01) of a cc. Typically, the total capacity or volume of the syringe determines the calibration. It is very important to count the number of spaces between each whole cc (or mL) to determine how a specific syringe is calibrated. The ordered dosage typically determines which syringe is appropriate for use. In some instances, however, the type of medication (insulin) determines the appropriate syringe to be used.

When reading the volume contained in a syringe, the syringe is held in the position indicated in the figure. The very top line marked on any syringe indicates zero and it is from this point downward that the volume is read. The black plunger may cause confusion. It has two distinct rings that are visibly in contact with the barrel of the syringe. The volume is read at the top of the uppermost ring where it contacts the barrel. This syringe reads 1.5 cc (or 1.5 mL).

The 3 cc syringe is the most widely used size of syringe because a high percentage of orders for medication falls in the 1–3 cc range. There are 10 calibrations per cc or mL; therefore, the syringe is calibrated in tenths and its total volume is 3 cc (3 mL).

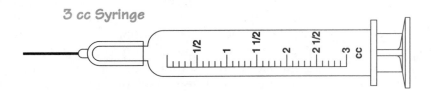

PREFILLED SYRINGE

Prefilled syringes are filled by the manufacturer with a standard single dosage of a specific medication. The syringe is clearly labeled as to the drug and dosage it contains. It is usually calibrated in tenths with a 2.5 cc (2.5 mL) total capacity. It is routinely overfilled by 0.1 to 0.2 cc to allow for the expulsion of air prior to injection. All excess medication contained in the syringe must be discarded before injection. The syringe usually has the capacity to accommodate another drug if combined dosages have been ordered. Prefilled syringes are to be used once and discarded.

TUBERCULIN SYRINGE

This syringe is used when very small doses (less than 1 mL) of medication must be administered. It has a total capacity of 1 cc (mL) and is calibrated in hundredths (0.01). Each tenth (0.1) is actually numbered on the syringe.

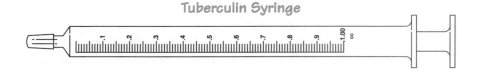

INSULIN SYRINGE

Insulin syringes are unique in that these syringes are used specifically to administer the insulin and must correspond directly to the dosage strength of the particular insulin. All insulin is measured and administered in Units. The most common strength of insulin, U-100, indicates that 100 Units of insulin are contained in a volume of 1 cc or mL.

Every insulin syringe will specify on the barrel of the syringe the strength of the insulin to be administered using that syringe. The typical U-100 syringe has a capacity of 1 cc (mL) with 100 calibrations, each representing 1 Unit (0.01 cc = 1 Unit). Another syringe is available for smaller doses of U-100 insulin. This syringe usually has a total capacity of 0.5 cc with 50 calibrations, each representing 1 Unit of insulin (again, 0.01 cc = 1 Unit). The smaller capacity makes the markings easier to read and ensures greater accuracy in the administration of the drug. Only in an emergency is insulin administered in anything other than an insulin syringe.

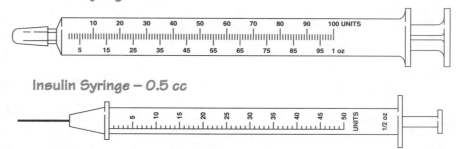

LARGE CAPACITY SYRINGES

When the dosage required exceeds 3 cc (mL), there are numerous syringes available. Syringes having capacities of 5, 6, 10, or 12 cc are calibrated in 2 tenths (0.2) of a cc. This means that they all have 5 divisions per whole cc. Each whole cc is numbered.

Syringes with capacities of 20 cc and above are calibrated in whole cc (mL) and numbered on the barrel of the syringe every 5th cc (mL). These syringes are only to be used to measure and administer large volumes.

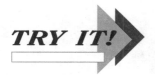

PRACTICE

Match the syringe with the standard calibration of that syringe.

_____ 1. 3 cc syringe   **A.** Units (0.01 cc = 1 Unit)

_____ 2. tuberculin syringe   **B.** tenths of a cc (0.1)

_____ 3. insulin syringe   **C.** 2 tenths of a cc (0.2)

_____ 4. 5, 6, 10, or 12 cc syringe   **D.** hundredths of a cc (0.01)

ANSWERS	
1. B	2. D
3. A	4. C

ADDITIONAL PRACTICE

Identify the utensils by name and volume, if appropriate.

5. _____

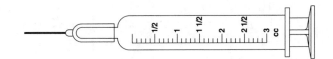

6. _____

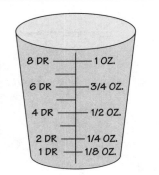

7. _____

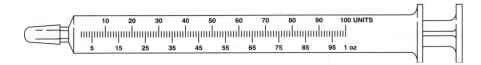

8. _____

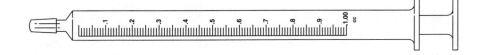

9. _____

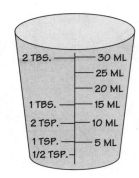

10. _____

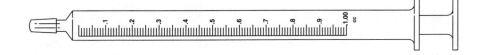

Identify the most appropriate syringe to be used to administer the following dosages.

_____ 11. 0.25 mL   **A.** tuberculin syringe
_____ 12. 1.3 cc   **B.** 3 cc syringe
_____ 13. 27 Units   **C.** insulin syringe
_____ 14. 2.4 cc   **D.** 10 cc syringe
_____ 15. 4.5 cc
_____ 16. 1.1 mL
_____ 17. 3.2 cc
_____ 18. 2.2 cc
_____ 19. 65 Units
_____ 20. 0.4 mL

Read the volume of medication that has been measured in the syringe.

21. _____   22. _____   23. _____   24. _____

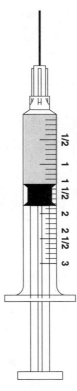
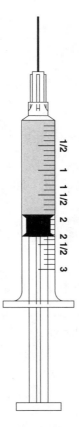
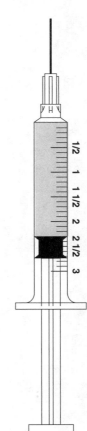
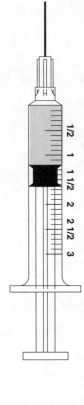

Indicate the following dosages by shading the syringe.

1. 0.45 cc

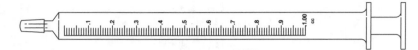

2. 80 Units U-100 insulin

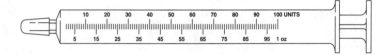

3. 2.4 cc

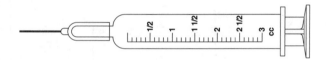

4. 7 mL

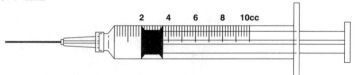

5. 0.75 cc

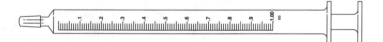

6. 0.33 mL

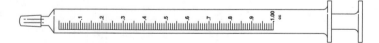

7. 2.1 mL

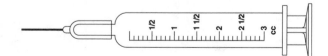

8. 2.5 cc

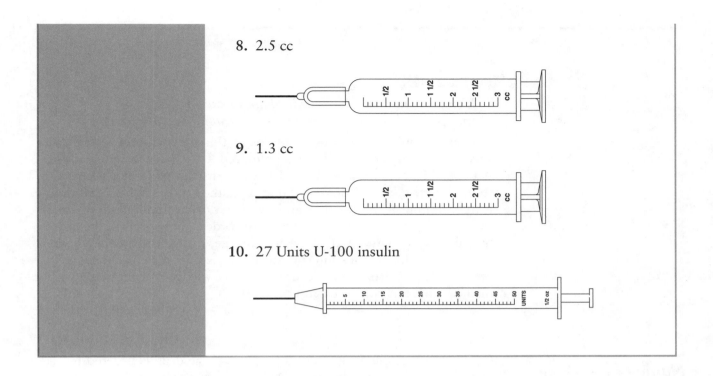

9. 1.3 cc

10. 27 Units U-100 insulin

OBJECTIVES

1. *Identify commonly used medical abbreviations.*
2. *Interpret a drug order which uses medical abbreviations.*

Every complete drug order contains all the information necessary to successfully deliver the medication required. It includes the name of the patient, the date and time the order was written, the name of the drug to be administered, the dosage of that drug, the route by which that drug is to be administered, the time and frequency of the administration, and the signature of the person that wrote the order. The aspects of the order that deal specifically with the drug, dosage, route, and frequency are often subject to further interpretation and sometimes calculation. In order to read a drug order accurately, a knowledge of commonly used medical abbreviations is essential.

Name of the Drug

The name of the drug appears first and if the drug is ordered by its trade or brand name, the first letter should be capitalized. A drug ordered by its generic name will normally not be capitalized.

Dosage of the Drug

The dosage of the drug is written in terms and abbreviations which are familiar from previous Units. Abbreviations referring to the solid or liquid form of the drug will follow the dosage.

COMMON FORM ABBREVIATIONS

ABBREVIATION	MEANING
tab	tablet
cap	capsule
elix	elixir
syr	syrup
sol	solution
ung	ointment

Route of Administration

The route of administration to be used will appear in abbreviated form immediately following the dosage ordered. These abbreviations must be memorized.

COMMON ROUTE ABBREVIATIONS

ABBREVIATIONS	MEANING
IM	intramuscular, within a muscle
IV	intravenous, within a vein
IV PB	intravenous piggyback
SC	subcutaneous, beneath the skin
po or PO	by mouth, orally
OD	right eye
OS	left eye
OU	both eyes
SL	sublingual, below the tongue
TOP	topical, applied to skin surface
R	rectally

Time and Frequency of Administration

Following the route by which the drug is to be administered, an abbreviation or set of abbreviations appear that clarify the administration by stating a specific time or the frequency with which the dosage is to be delivered.

COMMON FREQUENCY ABBREVIATIONS

ABBREVIATION		MEANING
a.c.	ac	before meals
p.c.	pc	after meals
ad. lib.	ad lib	freely, as desired
p.r.n.	prn	when necessary
h.s.	hs	hour of sleep, bedtime
stat		immediately
q.d.	qd	once a day, every day
q.o.d.	qod	every other day
b.i.d.	bid	twice a day
t.i.d.	tid	three times a day
q.i.d.	qid	four times a day
q.h.	qh	every hour
q.2h.	q2h	every 2 hours
q.3h.	q3h	every 3 hours
q.4h.	q4h	every 4 hours
q.6h.	q6h	every 6 hours
q.8h.	q8h	every 8 hours
q.12h.	q12h	every 12 hours

There are variations of these abbreviations. The periods may not always appear in the abbreviation and lowercase letters may be used instead of uppercase and vice versa, so it is extremely important that any confusion regarding the correct interpretation of the abbreviations be addressed to the original writer of the order.

Additional Descriptive Information

Abbreviations of certain common words frequently are used to shorten the drug order. Other abbreviations also appear which further describe and clarify the order.

GENERAL ABBREVIATIONS	
ABBREVIATION	**MEANING**
a	before
aa	of each
c	with
s	without
p	after
q	every
os	mouth
sos	if necessary
aq	water
NPO	nothing by mouth
rep	repeat
non rep	do not repeat

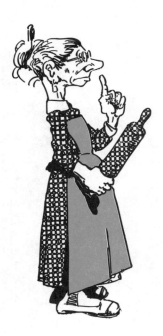

The abbreviation "non rep" means do not repeat.
I repeat, the abbreviation "non rep"...

Here's some typical information you might encounter and how you would interpret it.

NAME	DOSAGE	ROUTE	FREQUENCY	ADDITIONAL DESCRIPTION
A.				
Darvon-N	100 mg tab	PO	q.3-4h. p.r.n.	severe muscle pain
B.				
NPH insulin	25 Units	SC	q.d.	a.c. breakfast
C.				
aminophylline	0.5 g	R		stat non rep
D.				
nitroglycerin	0.4 mg tab	SL	p.r.n.	chest pain

Interpretation

A. Administer a 100-milligram tablet of Darvon-N by mouth every 3-4 hours as necessary for severe muscle pain.

B. Administer 25 Units of NPH insulin subcutaneously every day before breakfast.

C. Administer 0.5 gram of aminophylline rectally immediately and do not repeat.

D. Administer 0.4 milligram of nitroglycerin under the tongue as needed for chest pain.

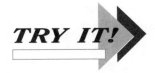

TRY IT!

PRACTICE

Read and interpret the drug orders.

1. morphine sulfate	15 mg	SC	q.4h.		
2. Tylenol	0.6 g	PO	q.4h.	p.r.n.	headache
3. atropine sulfate (optic) 1% sol	2 gtt	OD	q.d. t.i.d.		

ANSWERS

1. Administer 15 milligrams of morphine sulfate subcutaneously every 4 hours.
2. Administer 0.6 gram of Tylenol by mouth every 4 hours as necessary for headache.
3. Administer 2 drops of atropine sulfate 1% solution in the right eye every day three times a day.

ADDITIONAL PRACTICE

Interpret the following abbreviations.

4. SC _____   5. a.c. _____

6. stat _____   7. OS _____

8. ad.lib. _____   9. q.2h. _____

10. a _____   11. p _____

12. p.r.n. _____   13. q.o.d. _____

Write the appropriate abbreviation.

14. intramuscular _____   15. by mouth _____

16. both eyes _____   17. after meals _____

18. every hour _____   19. every 12 hours _____

20. before _____   21. tablet _____

22. without _____   23. once a day, every day _____

ON THE JOB

Interpret the following physician's orders.

1. phenylephrine HCl   0.12% sol   2 gtt   q. 3-4 h.

   _____

2. propoxyphene HCl   65 mg tab   q.4h.   p.r.n.

   _____

3. acetaminophen   500 mg   PO   q.4h   p.r.n.   headache

   _____

4. Demerol   75 mg   IM   q.4h   p.r.n.   pain

   _____

5. chlordiazepoxide HCl   5 mg tab   PO   q.i.d.

   _____

PART 3: READING DRUG LABELS

OBJECTIVES

1. *Identify and interpret specific information on a drug label.*
   A. *Generic and trade name of the drug*
   B. *Drug manufacturer*
   C. *Dosage strength*
   D. *Form of the drug*
   E. *Supply dosage*
   F. *Total volume of container*
   G. *Expiration date*
2. *Express the difference between dosage strength and supply dosage.*

The drug label on a medication contains information that is critical to the correct administration of the drug, such as generic and brand name manufacturer, dosage strength, form, total volume, directions for mixing powdered drugs, expiration date, and additional information.

Generic and Brand Name of the Drug

A drug label *must* identify the official (generic) name of the drug. The official national listing of drugs is the United States Pharmacopeia (USP). Initials indicating the USP may be used with the generic name and should not be confused with other abbreviations on the label. Some drug labels list only the generic name.

Most labels, however, identify a drug by two names. The other is the brand or trade name which is identified by ®, the registration symbol. A drug has only *one* official name, but different pharmaceutical companies register their own trade name for that drug. Drugs may be ordered by the generic (official) name or the trade (brand) name. The manufacturer of the drug is identified by name.

Dosage Strength (Weight of the Drug)

The dosage strength or weight of the drug is expressed on the label with a unit of measure such as grams, Units, mEq, or milligrams, for example, 0.5 mg, 250 U, 20 mEq, 1000 Units, and 100 mcg. Often, the dosage strength represents an average dosage that would be given to an average patient at one time. Occasionally, the dosage strength is listed in two systems of measurement such as: 0.6 mg (gr $\frac{1}{100}$) or 15 mg (gr $\frac{1}{4}$).

Combination drugs are preparations which contain a mixture of several drugs together. Often the dosage strength is not listed for combination drugs. They are ordered by tablet, by capsule, or by milliliter and not by dosage strength.

Form of the Drug

The drug may be in solid form (tablets, capsules, etc.) or liquid form. A tablet or capsule contains a certain weight of a drug. A volume of solution (usually stated in cc or mL) contains a certain weight of a drug.

Supply Dosage (On-hand Dosage)

The supply dosage or *on-hand dosage* is the dosage strength (weight) together with the form of the drug.

DOSAGE STRENGTH		FORM	SUPPLY DOSAGE (on-hand dosage)
Solid: 50 mg	in	1 tablet	50 mg/tablet
Liquid: 50 mg	in	1 cc	50 mg/cc
Solid: 200 mcg	in	1 capsule	200 mcg/capsule
Liquid: 200 mcg	in	5 mL	200 mcg/5 mL
Liquid: 100 mg	in	2 mL	100 mg/2 mL
Liquid: 1000 U	in	1 mL	1000 U/1 mL

The dosage ordered by the physician may be expressed in terms of weight only. The order may not state the number of milliliters (or cc) necessary to deliver that dosage.

Total Container Volume

The total number of milliliters (mL) or cubic centimeters (cc) in the container is listed on the label. Today, many tablets and capsules are packaged in unit dosages; that is, a single tablet or capsule in a blister pack. If the container holds multiple doses, however, the total number of tablets or capsules is identified.

Directions for Mixing or Reconstituting Powdered Drugs

Certain drugs that are supplied in powder form must be dissolved in a liquid before they can be administered. The directions for preparing solutions from powdered drugs may be printed on the drug label or may be included in the drug literature or inserts.

Expiration Date and Additional Information

The expiration date is the last date on which the drug should be used. Expiration may be abbreviated as EXP. Warnings regarding storage and the use of the drug are examples of other information which may be included on the label.

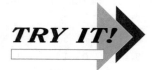

TRY IT!

PRACTICE

Identify each of the following as *dosage strength*, *form*, or *supply dosage*.

1. 0.5 mg _____
2. liquid (cc, mL, etc.) _____
3. gr $\frac{1}{75}$ _____
4. capsule _____
5. 1 mEq/mL _____
6. 500 mg per tablet _____

ADDITIONAL PRACTICE

Match the following lists.

_____ 7. Vistaril®	**A.** Expiration date
_____ 8. cc (liquid)	**B.** Drug manufacturer
_____ 9. 300,000 Units	**C.** Dosage strength
_____ 10. allopurinol	**D.** Form of the drug
_____ 11. The Upjohn Company	**E.** Trade (brand) name of drug
_____ 12. ampicillin	**F.** Supply dosage (on-hand dosage)
_____ 13. gr 1/100/tablet	**G.** Generic (official) name of drug
_____ 14. EXP 12/94	
_____ 15. 250 mcg/5 mL	
_____ 16. 4 mg	
_____ 17. 50 mg/cc	
_____ 18. Librium®	
_____ 19. 250 mcg/capsule	
_____ 20. capsule	
_____ 21. mL (liquid)	
_____ 22. digoxin	
_____ 23. tablet	
_____ 24. 60 mg/tablet	
_____ 25. Expires 2/94	
_____ 26. Parke-Davis	

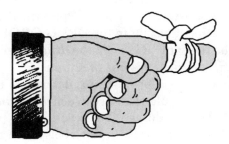

Remember: to calculate dosage you must know the desired dosage prescribed by the physician and the on-hand dosage which is available.

PART 4: PROPORTION DOSAGE

OBJECTIVES

1. *Given a supply dosage and a drug order, calculate oral drug dosages using proportion.*
2. *Determine the number of tablets or capsules necessary to deliver a prescribed dose.*
3. *Determine the volume of liquid necessary to deliver a prescribed dose (in solution form).*

Dosage calculations for oral drugs depend upon the drug order from the physician and the supply dosage which is available. The drug order and the supply dosage *must* be in the same measurement units before the correct number of tablets or the correct volume of liquid can be determined.

Oral Drug Preparations

Oral (by mouth) medication may be solid or liquid drug preparations. Solid drug preparations include capsules, scored tablets, tablets, and enteric-coated tablets. A certain weight of a drug is contained in a capsule or tablet.

A capsule cannot be broken. The drug is contained in a gelatin cover.

A scored tablet has an indentation where the tablet can be broken for a partial dosage.

A tablet that is not scored cannot be broken.

An enteric-coated tablet has a covering which delays the absorption of the drug until it reaches the small intestine.

When a medication is in liquid form, a certain weight of a drug is contained in a volume (cc, mL, tsp, gtt, etc.) of solution. Remember that a cubic centimeter and a milliliter are equal in volume (1 cc = 1 mL).

To calculate dosages, it is important to first consider two pieces of information:
1. **DRUG ORDER—desired dosage prescribed by the physician.**
2. **ON-HAND dosage—supply dosage (weight/form) of the drug which is available.**

Then it is necessary to calculate the volume of solution or number of tablets to be administered that will deliver the drug order.

Step 1: The units of weight in the DRUG ORDER and the ON-HAND dosage must be the same. *Convert the drug order to the units of the on-hand dosage, if the units are not the same.*

Step 2: Then, using a proportion, determine the correct number of tablets, capsules, cc, or mL necessary to deliver the ordered dosage. The first ratio is the ON-HAND dosage. The second ratio (with a missing term) is the DRUG ORDER. The order of the labels in the two ratios must match.

Dosage Calculation: Solid Drug

A. DRUG ORDER: cephalexin 500 mg
    ON-HAND DOSAGE: 250 mg capsule

How many capsules should be administered?

Step 1: Convert the drug order to on-hand weight units. (A conversion is not necessary in this case because the order and the on-hand dosage are both in milligrams.)

Step 2: Determine the number of capsules to be given. Set up a proportion with the on-hand dosage as the first ratio and the drug order as the second ratio.

ON-HAND		DRUG ORDER			
$\dfrac{250 \text{ mg}}{1 \text{ capsule}}$	$=$	$\dfrac{500 \text{ mg}}{X \text{ capsule}}$ OR	$\dfrac{250}{1}$	$=$	$\dfrac{500}{X}$

$$250\, X = 500$$
$$X = 2 \text{ capsules}$$

B. DRUG ORDER: phenobarbital gr ss
    ON-HAND DOSAGE: gr $\frac{1}{4}$ tablet

Step 1: Convert the drug order to on-hand weight units. A conversion is not necessary. The order and the on-hand dosage are both in grains.

Step 2: Determine the number of tablets to be given.

ON-HAND		DRUG ORDER			
$\dfrac{1/4 \text{ gr}}{1 \text{ tablet}}$	$=$	$\dfrac{1/2 \text{ gr}}{X \text{ tablet}}$ OR	$\dfrac{1/4}{1}$	$=$	$\dfrac{1/2}{X}$

$$1/4\, X = 1/2$$
$$X = 1/2 \div 1/4 \quad = (1/2)(4/1) = \quad 4/2$$
$$X = 2 \text{ tablets}$$

C. DRUG ORDER: nitroglycerin gr $\frac{1}{200}$
    ON-HAND DOSAGE: 0.3-mg tablet

Step 1: Convert the drug order to on-hand weight units (grains to milligrams).

EQUIVALENT		DRUG ORDER
$\dfrac{1 \text{ grain}}{60 \text{ milligrams}}$	$=$	$\dfrac{1/200 \text{ grain}}{X \text{ milligrams}}$

$$X = (1/200)(60)$$
$$X = 0.3 \text{ mg}$$

The drug order is equivalent to 0.3 mg.

Step 2: Determine the number of tablets to be given. The drug order is for 0.3 mg and the on-hand supply is a 0.3-mg tablet. Obviously, one tablet is to be administered.

ON-HAND		DRUG ORDER
$\dfrac{0.3 \text{ mg}}{1 \text{ tablet}}$	$=$	$\dfrac{0.3 \text{ mg}}{X \text{ tablet}}$

$0.3\,X$	$=$	0.3
X	$=$	1 tablet

D. DRUG ORDER: ampicillin 0.5 g
 ON-HAND DOSAGE: 250 mg capsule

Step 1: Convert drug order to on-hand weight units (grams to milligrams).

EQUIVALENT		DRUG ORDER				
$\dfrac{1000 \text{ mg}}{1 \text{ g}}$	$=$	$\dfrac{X \text{ mg}}{0.5 \text{ g}}$	OR	$\dfrac{1000}{1}$	$=$	$\dfrac{X}{0.5}$

X	$=$	$(0.5)(1000)$
X	$=$	500 mg

The drug order is equivalent to 500 mg.

Step 2: Determine the number of capsules to be given.

ON-HAND		DRUG ORDER				
$\dfrac{250 \text{ mg}}{1 \text{ capsule}}$	$=$	$\dfrac{500 \text{ mg}}{X \text{ capsules}}$	OR	$\dfrac{250}{1}$	$=$	$\dfrac{500}{X}$

$250\,X$	$=$	500
X	$=$	2 capsules

E. DRUG ORDER: triamcinolone 12 mg
 ON-HAND DOSAGE: 8 mg tablet (scored)

Step 1: Convert drug order to on-hand weight units, if necessary.
Step 2: Determine the number of tablets to be given.

ON-HAND		DRUG ORDER				
$\dfrac{8 \text{ mg}}{1 \text{ tablet}}$	$=$	$\dfrac{12 \text{ mg}}{X \text{ tablet}}$	OR	$\dfrac{8}{1}$	$=$	$\dfrac{12}{X}$
$8\,X$	$=$	12				
X	$=$	$12/8$	$=$	$1\ 1/2$ tablets		

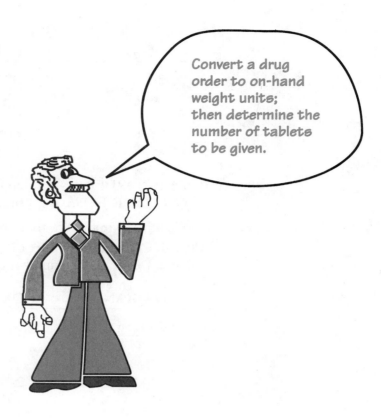

Convert a drug
order to on-hand
weight units;
then determine the
number of tablets
to be given.

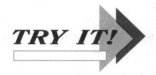
TRY IT!

PRACTICE

Find the correct number of capsules or tablets to be administered.

1. DRUG ORDER: tetracycline 0.75 g
    ON-HAND SUPPLY: 250 mg capsule
    _____ capsule

2. DRUG ORDER: meprobamate 200 mg
    ON-HAND SUPPLY: 400 mg tablet (scored)
    _____ tablet

ANSWERS

1. The drug order is for 750 mg which is supplied in 3 capsules.
2. 200 mg is delivered in $\frac{1}{2}$ tablet.

Dosage Calculation: Liquid Drug

A. DRUG ORDER: potassium chloride 30 mEq
    ON-HAND DOSAGE: oral solution 20 mEq/15 mL

How many milliliters are to be administered?

Step 1: Convert the drug order to on-hand weight units. (A conversion is not necessary in this case.)

Step 2: Determine the number of milliliters to be given. Set up a proportion with the on-hand supply as the first ratio and the drug order as the second ratio.

ON-HAND		DRUG ORDER				
$\dfrac{20 \text{ mEq}}{15 \text{ mL}}$	=	$\dfrac{30 \text{ mEq}}{X \text{ mL}}$	OR	$\dfrac{20}{15}$	=	$\dfrac{30}{X}$

$$20\,X = 450$$
$$X = 22.5 \text{ mL}$$

B. DRUG ORDER: erythromycin estolate 500 mg
ON-HAND DOSAGE: oral suspension 250 mg/5 ml

How many milliliters are to be administered?

Step 1: Convert drug order to on-hand weight units, if necessary.
Step 2: Determine the number of milliliters to be given.

ON-HAND		DRUG ORDER				
$\dfrac{250 \text{ mg}}{5 \text{ mL}}$	=	$\dfrac{500 \text{ mg}}{X \text{ mL}}$	OR	$\dfrac{250}{5}$	=	$\dfrac{500}{X}$

$$250\,X = 2500$$
$$X = 10 \text{ mL}$$

C. DRUG ORDER: phenobarbital gr ss
ON-HAND DOSAGE: elixir 15 mg/5 mL

Step 1: Convert drug order to on-hand weight units (grains to milligrams).

EQUIVALENT		DRUG ORDER				
$\dfrac{1 \text{ grain}}{60 \text{ mg}}$	=	$\dfrac{1/2 \text{ grain}}{X \text{ mg}}$	OR	$\dfrac{1}{60}$	=	$\dfrac{1/2}{X}$

$$X = (1/2)(60)$$
$$X = 30 \text{ mg}$$

The drug order is equivalent to 30 mg.

Step 2: Determine the number of milliliters to be given.

ON-HAND		DRUG ORDER				
$\dfrac{15 \text{ mg}}{5 \text{ mL}}$	=	$\dfrac{30 \text{ mg}}{X \text{ mL}}$	OR	$\dfrac{15}{5}$	=	$\dfrac{30}{X}$

$$15\,X = 150$$
$$X = 150/15 = 10 \text{ mL}$$

D. DRUG ORDER: cyclacillin 0.5 g
    ON-HAND DOSAGE: oral suspension 125 mg/5 mL

Step 1: Convert drug order to on-hand weight units (grams to milligrams).

EQUIVALENT		DRUG ORDER				
$\dfrac{1000 \text{ mg}}{1 \text{ g}}$	$=$	$\dfrac{X \text{ mg}}{0.5 \text{ g}}$	OR	$\dfrac{1000}{1}$	$=$	$\dfrac{X}{0.5}$

$$X = (0.5)(1000)$$
$$X = 500 \text{ mg}$$

Step 2: Determine the number of milliliters to be given.

ON-HAND		DRUG ORDER				
$\dfrac{125 \text{ mg}}{5 \text{ mL}}$	$=$	$\dfrac{500 \text{ mg}}{X \text{ mL}}$	OR	$\dfrac{125}{5}$	$=$	$\dfrac{500}{X}$

$$125 \, X = 2500$$
$$X = 2500/125 = 20 \text{ mL}$$

E. DRUG ORDER: promethazine HCl 25 mg
    ON-HAND DOSAGE: syrup 6.25 mg/teaspoon

Step 1: Convert drug order to on-hand weight units, if necessary.
Step 2: Determine the number of teaspoons to be given.

ON-HAND		DRUG ORDER				
$\dfrac{6.25 \text{ mg}}{1 \text{ teaspoon}}$	$=$	$\dfrac{25 \text{ mg}}{X \text{ teaspoon}}$	OR	$\dfrac{6.25}{1}$	$=$	$\dfrac{25}{X}$

$$6.25 \, X = 25$$
$$X = 25/6.25 = 4 \text{ teaspoons} \ (4 \text{ tsp} = 20 \text{ mL})$$

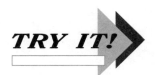

TRY IT!

PRACTICE

Find the correct volume of solution to be administered.

1. DRUG ORDER: phenobarbital gr $\frac{1}{3}$
   ON-HAND DOSAGE: elixir 20 mg/mL
      _____ mL

2. DRUG ORDER: methenamine 1 g
   ON-HAND DOSAGE: oral suspension 500 mg/5 mL
      _____ mL

ADDITIONAL PRACTICE

Write the number of tablets of allopurinol to be administered for each drug order.

ON-HAND DOSAGE: allopurinol 100-mg tablet (scored)

DRUG ORDER

3. allopurinol   0.2 g   _____

4. allopurinol   300 mg   _____

5. allopurinol   gr v   _____

6. allopurinol   0.15 g   _____

7. allopurinol   100 mg   _____

8. allopurinol   250 mg   _____

Write the volume of liquid theophylline to be administered for each drug order.

ON-HAND DOSAGE: liquid theophylline 150 mg/15 mL

DRUG ORDER

9. theophylline   0.05 g   _____

10. theophylline   150 mg   _____

11. theophylline   200 mg   _____

12. theophylline   0.15 g   _____

13. theophylline   100 mg   _____

14. theophylline   50 mg   _____

1. The drug order is nafcillin, 0.5 g. The dosage supply is 250 mg capsules. How many capsules should be administered? _____

2. The supply dosage (on-hand) is 5 grains per tablet. The physician orders 600 mg. How many tablets should be given? _____

3. The supply dosage (on-hand) is an elixir of 10 mg/5 mL, but 40 mg of a drug is ordered. How many mL should be administered? _____

4. The order is for 60 mg of Tylenol. The drug on-hand is 240 mg/10 mL. How many mL should be given? _____

5. The doctor's order is written for gr ii of a drug. The supply dosage (on-hand) is 240 mg half-scored tablets. How many tablets should be given? _____

6. A patient is to receive 300 mg of a pain reliever. The supply bottle contains 200 mg scored tablets. How many tablets should the patient be given? _____

7. The physician ordered 50 mcg of Drug R for the patient. The supply bottle contains 0.025 mg tablets. How many tablets are to be administered? _____

8. The on-hand supply of a drug is 100 mg tablets. How many tablets will deliver 0.1 g? _____

9. If the supply dosage is gr S/10 mL, how many milliliters would be administered for a 600 mg drug order? _____

10. Chloral hydrate, 500 mg, was ordered for the patient. The on-hand chloral hydrate syrup is labeled 250 mg/5 mL. How many milliliters are to be administered to the patient? _____

PART 5: PARENTERAL DOSAGE

OBJECTIVES

1. *Given a supply dosage and a drug order, calculate parenteral drug dosages using proportion.*
2. *Determine the volume of liquid necessary to deliver a prescribed dose (in solution form).*

Parenteral medications are administered to the body in a way other than the digestive tract. Dosage calculations for parenteral solutions follow the same procedure as dosage calculations for oral solutions. It is necessary to calculate the volume required to deliver a given drug order.

---◆◆

Parenteral Medication

These medications may be supplied in a liquid form that is contained in vials, ampules, or prefilled syringes. Other parenteral medications are supplied in a powder form which must be dissolved in a liquid, according to instructions.

These liquid parenteral medications are administered by injection. The most frequently used routes of administration are intramuscular (IM), subcutaneous (S.C.), and intravenous (IV).

It is difficult for more than 3 mL to be absorbed at one injection site. Therefore, most IM and S.C. solutions have been prepared so that the average IM or S.C. dosage is contained in a volume ranging from 1 to 3 mL. Most IM and S.C. dosages are prepared using a 3 cc syringe. Dosages that are contained in volumes of less than 1 cc may be prepared most accurately in a 1 cc tuberculin syringe.

Supply dosages (weight/volume) listed on parenteral drug labels may be expressed in metric, apothecary, ratio, and percentage strengths (1 cc and 1 mL are used interchangeably). Here are some examples.

SUPPLY DOSAGE (ON-HAND) IN METRIC AND APOTHECARY STRENGTH

20 mL = 80 mg	80 mg contained in 20 mL
1 mg = 5 cc	1 mg contained in 5 cc
1 mL = 250,000 Units	250,000 U contained in 1 mL
40 mEq/20 mL	40 mEq contained in 20 mL
1000 U/mL	1000 Units contained in 1 mL
25 mg/50 mL	25 mg contained in 50 mL
gr 1/4/cc	1/4 grain contained in 1 cc
100 mg/2 cc	100 mg contained in 2 cc

SUPPLY DOSAGE (ON-HAND) IN RATIO AND PERCENTAGE STRENGTH

50%	50 g/100 mL = 1 g/2 mL = 1000 mg/2 mL = 500 mg/1 mL
2%	2 g/100 mL = 1 g/50 mL = 1000 mg/50 mL = 20 mg/1 mL
1:1000	1 g/1000 mL = 1000 mg/1000 mL = 1 mg/1 mL
1:2000	1 g/2000 mL = 1000 mg/2000 mL = 1 mg/2 mL

Dosages that are ordered by ratio or percentage strength are generally requested by the number of cc or mL to be administered. In this case, it is not necessary to calculate the volume required to deliver a dosage, because it is already given.

DRUG ORDER: dextrose 50%   20 mL
SUPPLY DOSAGE: dextrose 50%

The volume (20 mL) to be diluted for the IV administration is stated in the drug order.

DRUG ORDER: epinephrine 1:1000   0.5 mL
SUPPLY DOSAGE: epinephrine 1:1000

The volume (0.5 mL) necessary to deliver the prescribed dosage is stated in the drug order.

Parenteral Dosage Calculation

Dosage calculations for parenteral solutions follow the same procedure as dosage calculations for oral solutions.

When the correct volume has been determined for an IM or S.C. dosage, it is administered by syringe. The IV dosage, however, is then diluted according to the physician's order or the manufacturer's instructions. This means that the IV dosage is added to an IV solution. IV dosages are delivered in IV solutions at a flow rate that is usually calculated in mL/hr or gtt/min. Flow rate calculations for IV fluids and medications are covered later in this unit.

When calculating parenteral dosages, round the answer to the closest amount that can be measured by the appropriate syringe. If the syringe is calibrated in tenths (such as a 3 cc syringe), round the calculation to the nearest tenth. If the syringe is calibrated in hundredths (1 cc tuberculin syringe), round the calculation to the nearest hundredth. The following examples involve dosage calculation only, not flow rates.

A. DRUG ORDER: morphine sulfate 15 mg
      SUPPLY DOSAGE: morphine sulfate 15 mg/mL

Step 1: Convert drug order to supply dosage units, if necessary.
Step 2: Determine volume necessary to deliver the drug order.

SUPPLY DOSAGE		DRUG ORDER			
$\dfrac{15 \text{ mg}}{1 \text{ mL}}$	$=$	$\dfrac{15 \text{ mg}}{X \text{ mL}}$	OR	$\dfrac{15}{1}$ $=$	$\dfrac{15}{X}$
15 X	$=$	15			
X	$=$	15/15	$=$	1 mL (1 cc)	

B. DRUG ORDER: sodium thiosalicylate 75 mg
SUPPLY DOSAGE: sodium thiosalicylate 50 mg/mL

Step 1: Convert drug order to supply dosage units, if necessary.
Step 2: Determine volume necessary to deliver drug order (75 mg).

SUPPLY DOSAGE	DRUG ORDER		
$\dfrac{50 \text{ mg}}{1 \text{ mL}}$ =	$\dfrac{75 \text{ mg}}{X \text{ mL}}$ OR	$\dfrac{50}{1}$ =	$\dfrac{75}{X}$

$$50 \, X = 75$$
$$X = 75/50 = 1.5 \text{ mL (1.5 cc)}$$

C. DRUG ORDER: atropine sulfate gr $\frac{1}{400}$
SUPPLY DOSAGE: atropine sulfate 0.4 mg per mL

Step 1: Convert drug order to supply dosage units (grains to milligrams).

(1 gr = 60 mg)

EQUIVALENT	DRUG ORDER		
$\dfrac{1 \text{ grain}}{60 \text{ mg}}$ =	$\dfrac{1/400 \text{ grain}}{X \text{ mg}}$ OR	$\dfrac{1}{60}$ =	$\dfrac{1/400}{X}$

$$X = 1/400(60) = 0.15 \text{ mg}$$

The drug order is for gr $\frac{1}{400}$ or 0.15 mg.

Step 2: Determine volume necessary to deliver drug order (0.15 mg).

SUPPLY DOSAGE	DRUG ORDER		
$\dfrac{0.4 \text{ mg}}{1 \text{ mL}}$ =	$\dfrac{0.15 \text{ mg}}{X \text{ mL}}$ OR	$\dfrac{0.4}{1}$ =	$\dfrac{0.15}{X}$

$$0.4 \, X = 0.15$$
$$X = 0.15/0.4 = 0.375 \text{ mL} \sim 0.38 \text{ mL}$$

The volume (less than 1 cc) would be measured in a 1 cc tuberculin syringe which is calibrated in hundredths. Round 0.375 to the nearest hundredth.

D. DRUG ORDER: fentanyl citrate 0.1 mg
SUPPLY DOSAGE: fentanyl citrate 250 mcg/5 mL

Step 1: Convert drug order to supply dosage units (milligrams to micrograms).

EQUIVALENT		DRUG ORDER				
$\dfrac{1000 \text{ mcg}}{1 \text{ mg}}$	=	$\dfrac{X \text{ mcg}}{0.1 \text{ mg}}$	OR	$\dfrac{1000}{1}$	=	$\dfrac{X}{0.1}$

$$X = 0.1(1000)$$
$$X = 100 \text{ mcg}$$

Step 2: Determine volume necessary to deliver drug order (100 mcg).

SUPPLY DOSAGE		DRUG ORDER				
$\dfrac{250 \text{ mcg}}{5 \text{ mL}}$	=	$\dfrac{100 \text{ mcg}}{X \text{ mL}}$	OR	$\dfrac{250}{5}$	=	$\dfrac{100}{X}$

250 X	=	5(100)	=	500
X	=	500/250	=	2 mL (2 cc)

E. DRUG ORDER: aminophylline 0.25 g
SUPPLY DOSAGE: aminophylline 500 mg/20 mL

Step 1: Convert drug order to supply dosage units (grams to milligrams).

EQUIVALENT		DRUG ORDER				
$\dfrac{1000 \text{ mg}}{1 \text{ g}}$	=	$\dfrac{X \text{ mg}}{0.25 \text{ g}}$	OR	$\dfrac{1000}{1}$	=	$\dfrac{X}{0.25}$

$$X = 250 \text{ mg}$$

Step 2: Determine the volume necessary to deliver drug order (250 mg).

SUPPLY DOSAGE		DRUG ORDER				
$\dfrac{500 \text{ mg}}{20 \text{ mL}}$	=	$\dfrac{250 \text{ mg}}{X \text{ mL}}$	OR	$\dfrac{500}{20}$	=	$\dfrac{250}{X}$

500 X	=	250(20)	=	5000
X	=	5000/500	=	10 mL

F. DRUG ORDER: heparin sodium 4500 Units
   SUPPLY DOSAGE: heparin sodium 10,000 Units/mL

Step 1: Convert drug order to supply dosage units, if necessary.
Step 2: Determine volume necessary to deliver drug order (4500 Units).

SUPPLY DOSAGE	DRUG ORDER

$$\frac{10{,}000 \text{ Units}}{1 \text{ mL}} = \frac{4500 \text{ Units}}{X \text{ mL}} \quad \text{OR} \quad \frac{10{,}000}{1} = \frac{4500}{X}$$

$$10{,}000 \ X = 4500$$
$$X = 4500/10{,}000 = 0.45 \text{ mL} \ (0.45 \text{ cc})$$

G. DRUG ORDER: potassium chloride 20 mEq
   SUPPLY DOSAGE: potassium chloride 2 mEq/mL

Step 1: Convert drug order to supply dosage units, if necessary.
Step 2: Determine volume necessary to deliver drug order (20 mEq).

SUPPLY DOSAGE	DRUG ORDER

$$\frac{2 \text{ mEq}}{1 \text{ mL}} = \frac{20 \text{ mEq}}{X \text{ mL}} \quad \text{OR} \quad \frac{2}{1} = \frac{20}{X}$$

$$2 \ X = 20$$
$$X = 10 \text{ mL} \ (10 \text{ cc})$$

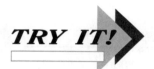

PRACTICE

Determine the volume necessary to deliver the given drug order.

SUPPLY DOSAGE: meperidine   50 mg = 1 mL

1. **DRUG ORDER:**   meperidine   100 mg   _____
2. **DRUG ORDER:**   meperidine   75 mg   _____

ANSWERS

1. 2 mL or 2 cc
2. 1.5 mL or 1.5 cc

ADDITIONAL PRACTICE

Calculate the amount of solution necessary to obtain the drug order.

SUPPLY DOSAGE: atropine sulfate   0.4 mg/mL

   3. DRUG ORDER: 0.001 g   _____

   4. DRUG ORDER: 0.15 mg   _____

   5. DRUG ORDER: gr $\frac{1}{300}$ _____

   6. DRUG ORDER: 0.0004 g   _____

   7. DRUG ORDER: 0.3 mg   _____

   8. DRUG ORDER: gr $\frac{1}{100}$ _____

   9. DRUG ORDER: 1 mg   _____

10. DRUG ORDER: 0.2 mg   _____

11. DRUG ORDER: 0.6 mg   _____

12. DRUG ORDER: gr $\frac{1}{150}$ _____

ON THE JOB

1. The digoxin vial is labeled 0.25 mg = 1 cc. The physician orders digoxin 0.15 mg. How many milliliters are equivalent to 0.15 mg? _____

2. A physician orders 250 mg of a drug. The vial is labeled 1 g/mL. How many cc should be administered? _____

3. A vial is labeled meperidine HCl 50 mg = 1 cc. The physician orders 40 mg. How many cc are to be injected? _____

4. The supply dosage of heparin sodium is 1000 Units/mL. Calculate the volume necessary to provide the dosage ordered. _____
   DRUG ORDER: 700 Units

5. A physician orders 15 mEq. The dosage on hand is 2 mEq/mL. What volume contains the prescribed dosage? _____

PART 6: PEDIATRIC DOSAGES

OBJECTIVES

1. *Read a nomogram to determine body surface area (BSA).*
2. *Use a child's body weight or body surface area (BSA) to calculate a pediatric dosage.*
3. *Calculate pediatric dosages based on recommended usual doses using a formula or a proportion.*

Pediatric dosages are less than adult dosages. Infants and children differ from adults in height, weight, body surface area, and metabolism. They need less medication than adults to achieve a desired effect. Administering an incorrect dosage to an adult is very dangerous. Administering an incorrect dosage to a child is even more dangerous. It is imperative to first make sure that the prescribed dosage is a safe and correct dosage. However, underdosage can at times be as dangerous as overdosage.

Pediatric Dosage Overview

Drug labels and inserts provide critical information regarding pediatric dosages. Calculations shown here are based on the drug manufacturer's recommendations, not the drug order. The correct dosage according to the drug recommendations should be compared to the drug order to ensure that the drug was correctly prescribed.

Calculating the correct dosage for an infant or child is accomplished in several steps. It is necessary to determine dosage recommendations from the drug label or drug literature. The usual dosage is most often expressed in terms of the child's body weight, such as mg/kg or mg/lb. Check carefully to see if the recommended dosage is specified as a *total daily dosage* or as a *single dose*. A total daily dosage must be divided by the number of doses to be administered. A range of milligrams/weight (such as 20-40 mg/kg) may be listed, depending on the condition of the child or the severity of the illness.

Pediatric Dosage Based on Weight

The pediatric dosage calculation based on a weight recommendation can be done using a proportion or simple multiplication. Multiply the usual dose times the weight of the child. The weight of the child must be expressed in the same units as the manufacturer's recommendation.

CHILD'S DOSAGE = RECOMMENDED DOSE **x** CHILD'S WEIGHT

OR

$$\text{CHILD'S DOSAGE} = \frac{mg}{kg} \times \text{CHILD'S WEIGHT (kg)}$$

OR

$$\text{CHILD'S DOSAGE} = \frac{mg}{lb} \times \text{CHILD'S WEIGHT (lb)}$$

A. Calculate a recommended dosage for a 45 pound child.

Recommended usual dose: Children under 50 pounds, 50 mg/kg/day in divided doses q6h.

    1. Express the weight in kilograms, rounded to the nearest tenth.
        45 pounds/2.2 ~   20.5 kg

    2. Determine the recommended *total daily dosage* for a 20.5 kg child.

Using Multiplication:

$$\text{CHILD'S DOSAGE} = \frac{50 \text{ mg}}{1 \text{ kg}} \times 20.5 \text{ kg} = \frac{1025}{1} = 1025 \text{ mg}$$

Using Proportion:

USUAL DOSAGE/WT.

$$\frac{50 \text{ mg}}{1 \text{ kg}} = \frac{X}{20.5 \text{ kg}} \quad \text{OR} \quad \frac{50}{1} = \frac{X}{20.5}$$

$$X = 50(20.5) = 1025$$

The *total daily recommended dosage* for a 20.5 kg child is 1025 mg.

    3. The *total daily dosage* is to be administered *in divided doses*, every 6 hours.
        24 hr/6 hr   =   4 times per day

TOTAL DAILY DOSAGE/NUMBER OF DOSES   =   SINGLE DOSE
    1025/4   ~   256 mg

B. An initial recommended dose for an infant is 15 mg/kg. The infant weighs 4000 g. How many milligrams should be administered in the initial dose? If the supply dosage is 500 mg/10 mL, what volume contains the initial dose?

    1. The weight must be expressed in kilograms.
        4000 g/1000 g   =   4 kg

    2. Determine the number of milligrams in the initial dose.

Using Multiplication:

$$\text{CHILD'S DOSAGE} = \frac{15 \text{ mg}}{1 \text{ kg}} \times 4 \text{ kg} = \frac{60}{1} = 60 \text{ mg}$$

Using Proportion:

USUAL DOSAGE/WT.

$$\frac{15 \text{ mg}}{1 \text{ kg}} = \frac{X}{4 \text{ kg}} \quad \text{OR} \quad \frac{15}{1} = \frac{X}{4}$$

$$X = 4(15) = 60 \text{ mg}$$

3. Determine the volume that contains the initial dose of 60 mg.

$$\frac{500 \text{ mg}}{10 \text{ mL}} \quad = \quad \frac{60 \text{ mg}}{X \text{ mL}} \qquad \text{OR} \qquad \frac{500}{10} = \frac{60}{X}$$

$$500 \text{ X} \quad = \quad 10(60) \quad = \quad 600$$
$$\text{X} \quad = \quad 600/500 \quad = \quad 1.2 \text{ mL}$$

C. Calculate the recommended *single dose* range for a 17 pound infant
Information regarding usual dosage:
20-40 mg/kg/day in divided doses every 8 hours

   1. The weight of the infant must be expressed in kilograms, rounded to the nearest tenth.
     17/2.2   ~   7.7 kg
     The 17 pound child weighs approximately 7.7 kg.

   2. The *total daily dosage range* must be expressed in milligrams.

Using Multiplication:

$$\text{CHILD'S DOSAGE} = \quad \frac{20 \text{ mg}}{1 \text{ kg}} \quad \times \quad 7.7 \quad = \quad 154 \text{ mg}$$

$$\text{CHILD'S DOSAGE} = \quad \frac{40 \text{ mg}}{1 \text{ kg}} \quad \times \quad 7.7 \quad = \quad 308 \text{ mg}$$

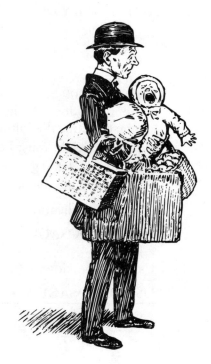

I guarantee you. This baby's BSA is primarily WET!

Using Proportion:

$$\frac{20 \text{ mg}}{1 \text{ kg}} = \frac{X}{7.7 \text{ kg}} \qquad\qquad \frac{40 \text{ mg}}{1 \text{ kg}} = \frac{X}{7.7 \text{ kg}}$$

$$X = 20(7.7) = 154 \text{ mg} \qquad X = 40(7.7) = 308 \text{ mg}$$

The total daily dosage range for a 7.7 kg infant is 154 mg-308 mg, depending on the child's age and severity of the illness.

3. A dose every 8 hours is given 3 times per day.
    24 hours/8 hours   =   3 times per day

4. The single dose is the total daily dosage divided into 3 equal parts.
    154/3   ~   51.3 mg
    308/3   ~   102.7 mg

The single dose range for a 7.7 kg infant is 51.3 mg-102.7 mg.

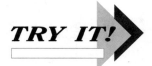
TRY IT!

PRACTICE

Calculate a recommended dose in mg for each child.
Recommended USUAL DOSE: 10 mg/kg

1. Child A: 33 lb   _____

2. Child B: 10 kg   _____

ANSWERS
1. 150 mg
2. 100 mg

Pediatric Dosage Based on Body Surface Area

Dosage calculations for infants and children up to the age of 12 can also be accomplished using the Body Surface Area (BSA) method. Body Surface Area (BSA) is expressed in square meters (m^2). A chart called the nomogram is used to estimate the BSA necessary for dosage calculations.

Height and weight together can be used to determine BSA from the nomogram. If an infant or child is of normal height and weight, the BSA can be determined using weight alone. When connecting height and weight with a ruler, or just indicating the weight in the enclosed area, pay special attention to the calibration between numbers. It should be noted that the calibrations are not consistent from the top to the bottom of the graph.

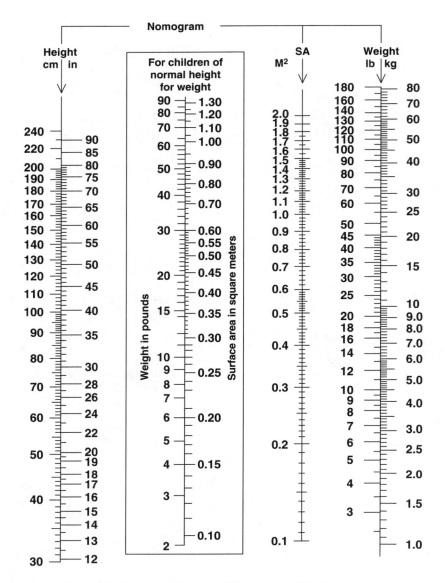

Nomogram

Height
cm | in

**For children of
normal height
for weight**

Weight in pounds

Surface area in square meters

SA
M²

Weight
lb | kg

Reprinted with permission from R.E. Behman and V.C. Vaughan,
Nelson Textbook of Pediatrics, 12th edition. Philadelphia, W.B.
Saunders Co. 1987.

Use a ruler to connect the height (extreme left) and weight (extreme right) of the child. Read the BSA in m² where the ruler intersects the SA graph. Or, for children of normal height and weight, locate the weight in the graph below and read the BSA from within the enclosure.

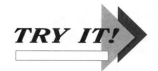

TRY IT!

PRACTICE

Indicate the BSA in m², using the nomogram.

1. Child is 110 cm and 50 lb _____

2. Child is 64 cm and 6.8 kg _____

3. Child is 30 in tall and weighs 26 lb _____

Indicate the BSA in m² for a child of normal height and weight.

4. Child weighs 15 pounds _____

5. Child weighs 15 kg _____

ANSWERS		
1. 0.84 m²	**2.** 0.36 m²	**3.** 0.52 m²
4. 0.36 m²	**5.** 0.64 m²	

Using BSA and Usual Children's Doses

Drug labels and drug literature often state usual children's dosages in terms of milligrams per square meter (mg/m²). The pediatric dosage calculation can be done using simple multiplication. Multiply the recommended dose/m² **x** the child's BSA.

CHILD'S DOSE = mg/m² x Child's BSA (m²)

Or, the dosage calculation can be accomplished using a proportion.

A. Calculate the correct children's dose. Recommended child's dose: 20 mg/m². The child has a BSA of 0.4 m².

Using Multiplication:

$$\text{CHILD'S DOSE} = \frac{20 \text{ mg}}{1 \text{ m}^2} \quad \text{x} \quad 0.4 \text{ m}^2 = 8 \text{ mg}$$

Using Proportion:

$$\frac{20 \text{ mg}}{1 \text{ m}^2} = \frac{X \text{ mg}}{0.4 \text{ m}^2} \quad \text{OR} \quad \frac{20}{1} = \frac{X}{0.4}$$

$$X = 20(0.4) = 8 \text{ mg}$$

B. Calculate the correct dosage range. Recommended child's dose: 25-40 mg/m². The child has a BSA of 0.78 m².

Using Multiplication:

$$\text{CHILD'S DOSE} = \frac{25 \text{ mg}}{1 \text{ m}^2} \quad \text{x} \quad 0.78 \text{ m}^2 = 19.5 \text{ mg}$$

$$\text{CHILD'S DOSE} = \frac{40 \text{ mg}}{1 \text{ m}^2} \quad \text{x} \quad 0.78 \text{ m}^2 = 31.2 \text{ mg}$$

The dosage range for a child with a BSA of 0.78 m² is 19.5 mg-31.2 mg.

Using Proportion:

$$\frac{25 \text{ mg}}{1 \text{ m}^2} = \frac{X \text{ mg}}{0.78 \text{ m}^2} \qquad \frac{40 \text{ mg}}{1 \text{ m}^2} = \frac{X \text{ mg}}{0.78 \text{ m}^2}$$

$$X = 25(0.78) = 19.5 \text{ mg} \qquad X = 40(0.78) = 31.2 \text{ mg}$$

Using BSA and Usual Adult Doses

A correct pediatric dose can be calculated using the child's BSA and the usual adult dose. The recommended average adult dose is based upon the average 140-lb adult having a BSA of 1.7 m².

A formula is used to determine the child's dose based on the adult's dose. The child's BSA is a fractional part of the adult's BSA, and the child's dose is a fractional part of the adult's dose. The child's BSA is expressed in m². The average BSA for the adult (1.7) is expressed in m².

$$\text{CHILD'S DOSE} = \frac{\text{Child's BSA (m}^2)}{1.7 \text{ m}^2} \times \text{ADULT DOSE}$$

A. The average adult dose is 500 mg. What is the dosage for a child whose BSA is 0.45 m²? Express the answer to the nearest tenth.

$$\text{CHILD'S DOSE} = \frac{\text{Child's BSA}}{1.7 \text{ m}^2} \times \text{ADULT DOSE}$$

$$= \frac{0.45}{1.7} \times 500 = \frac{225}{1.7} \sim 132.4 \text{ mg}$$

B. The average adult dose is 1500 Units. The child has a BSA of 0.65 m². What is the child's dosage, expressed to the nearest tenth?

$$\text{CHILD'S DOSE} = \frac{\text{Child's BSA (m}^2)}{1.7 \text{ m}^2} \times \text{ADULT DOSE}$$

$$= \frac{0.65}{1.7} \times 1500 \text{ Units} = \frac{97.5}{1.7} = 573.5 \text{ Units}$$

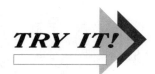

PRACTICE

Calculate the correct dosage for a child with a BSA of 0.45 m². Express answers to the nearest tenth.

1. Usual Child's Dosage: 25 mg/m²
2. Usual Child's Dosage: 35 mg/m²
3. Usual Adult Dosage: 60 Units
4. Usual Adult Dosage: 200 mg

ANSWERS

1. 11.3 mg   2. 15.8 mg   3. 15.9 Units   4. 52.9 mg

ADDITIONAL PRACTICE

Determine the BSA (from West's Nomogram) of each child.

	HEIGHT	WEIGHT	
5.	148 cm	40 kg	_____
6.	30 in	25 lb	_____
7.	80 in	10 kg	_____
8.	Child of normal height and weight.		
		10 lb	_____
9.	Child of normal height and weight.		
		25 lb	_____

Calculate the correct *single* pediatric dose based on weight. Round calculations to the nearest tenth.
Usual Child's Dose: 2.5 mg/lb q.i.d.

10.	Weight of the child:	25 lb	_____ mg
11.	Weight of the child:	18 kg	_____ mg
12.	Weight of the child:	25 kg	_____ mg

Calculate the correct *single* pediatric dose based on weight.
Usual Child's Dose: 40 mg/kg/day in equally divided doses q6h
Round the weight to the nearest tenth kilogram.

13.	Weight of the child:	26 lb	_____ mg
14.	Weight of the child:	18.5 kg	_____ mg

Calculate the correct pediatric dosage for a child with a BSA (body surface area) of 0.65 m^2. Round to the nearest tenth, if necessary.

15.	Usual Child's Dosage:	30 mg/m^2	_____ mg
16.	Usual Child's Dosage:	45 mg/m^2	_____ mg
17.	Usual Adult Dosage:	10 mg	_____ mg
18.	Usual Adult Dosage:	1500 Units	_____ Units
19.	Usual Adult Dosage:	100 mg	_____ mg

A child weighs 20 kg and is 110 cm tall.
Recommended CHILD'S DOSE: 250 mg/m^2 IV q8h
SUPPLY DOSAGE: 50 mg/mL

1. Using West's nomogram, what is the BSA of this child? _____

2. Based on the recommended dose, how many milligrams are to be given every 8 hours? _____

3. What volume of medication contains the proper dosage? (This volume must be diluted in the proper solution before the IV can be administered.) Round to the nearest tenth. _____

A child's BSA is 0.55 m^2 and he weighs 27 pounds.
Usual CHILD'S DOSE: 20 mg/kg/day p.o. in divided doses tid
SUPPLY DOSAGE: 125 mg/5 mL

4. What is the weight of the child in kilograms? Round to the nearest tenth. _____

5. What is the total daily dosage in milligrams? Round to the nearest tenth. _____

6. What is a single dose in milligrams? Round to the nearest tenth. _____

7. What volume of medication contains a single dose? Round to the nearest tenth. _____

A child's BSA is 0.72 m^2
Usual ADULT DOSE: 50 mg q4h
SUPPLY DOSAGE: 50 mg/mL

8. What is a single pediatric dose in milligrams? Round to the nearest tenth. _____

9. What volume is necessary to deliver the correct pediatric dose? Round to the nearest hundredth. _____

10. The child's BSA is 0.42 m^2. The adult dosage is 35 Units. Calculate the normal pediatric dosage rounded to the nearest whole Unit. _____

PART 7: INTRAVENOUS FLUID FLOW RATE CALCULATION

OBJECTIVES

1. *Express the flow rate of IV fluids in milliliters per hour based on the physician's order.*
2. *Recognize the calibration (drop factor) of an IV administration set.*
3. *Convert milliliter per hour to a flow rate expressed in drops per minute using a formula.*

The administration of intravenous fluids and medications requires the utmost care and precision. It is especially important to pay attention to time units, such as minutes and hours, and make sure the units are expressed properly when using the formula.

IV Flow Rates

The prescribed solutions are infused at a certain rate. The flow rate is a volume of fluid that is delivered per unit of time. Physicians' orders (in mL/hr or mL/min) can be converted to gtt/min (flow rate).

In order to calculate the rate of flow, it is necessary to know three pieces of information:

1. **The volume of fluid to be infused (in mL or cc).**
2. **The amount of time for the infusion.**
3. **The drop factor calibration (gtt/mL) of the administration set, specified on the package.**

Drop size depends upon the size of the IV tubing. Since all tubing is not the same size, each manufacturer specifies the number of drops that deliver 1 mL (or 1 cc) of fluid. (Recall that 1 mL = 1 cc.) This calibration in gtt/mL or gtt/cc is called the drop factor. The drop factor calibration of the administration set is needed to calculate flow rates.

A standard macrodrip set may have a drop factor calibration of 10 gtt/mL, 15 gtt/mL, or 20 gtt/mL, depending on the design of the tubing. These sets are used in routine adult IV administrations.

A microdrip set (which is used when more exact measurements are needed) is calibrated at 60 gtt/mL (60 gtt/cc). These sets are routinely used in pediatric and intensive care units.

The physician most frequently orders intravenous (IV) fluids to be administered in terms of mL/hr (or cc/hr). Medications contained in smaller volumes of fluid may also be ordered in terms of mL/min. The prescribed volume is to be administered in a specified time period. This is accomplished by adjusting the rate at which the IV runs (or infuses). The mL/hr or mL/min orders are converted to a flow rate expressed in gtt/min.

**Use two steps to calculate the flow rate in drops per minute (gtt/min).
In the calculations, round mL, cc, and gtt to the nearest whole.**

1. Determine mL/hr (or cc/hr). Divide the total volume to be infused by the number of hours allowed for the infusion.

$$mL/hr = \frac{\text{Total volume (mL) to be administered}}{\text{Total number of hours to be infused}}$$

2. Determine the flow rate in gtt/min. Multiply the volume (mL/hr) to be infused by the drop factor of the administration set. Divide that product by 60 minutes.

$$\frac{\text{(mL/hr) (gtt Factor)}}{60 \text{ minutes}} = \text{gtt/min}$$

Steps 1 and 2 can be combined to calculate the rate (R) as follows:

$$R = \frac{\text{Total volume (mL) X drop factor (gtt)}}{\text{hours X minutes}}$$

A. A patient is to receive an IV of 1000 mL to run over 8 hours. The tubing set is calibrated at 10 gtt/mL. Calculate the flow rate in gtt/min.

1. Determine mL/hr.

$$\frac{\text{Total volume (mL)}}{\text{Total time (hr)}} = \frac{1000}{8} = 125 \text{ mL/hr}$$

Determine the gtt/min necessary to deliver 125 mL/hr.

$$\frac{\text{(mL/hr) (drop factor)}}{60 \text{ minutes}} = \frac{(125)(10)}{60} = \frac{1250}{60} \sim 21 \text{ gtt/min}$$

B. The physician orders an IV of 50 mL to infuse in 40 minutes using a set calibration at 60 gtt/mL. Calculate the flow rate in gtt/min.

1. Determine mL/hr. (40 minutes is a fractional part of an hour, $\frac{40}{60} = \frac{2}{3}$ hr)

$$\frac{\text{Total volume (mL)}}{\text{Total time (hr)}} = \frac{50 \text{ mL}}{2/3 \text{ hr}} = \frac{50}{2/3} = 50 (3/2) = \frac{150}{2} = 75 \text{ mL/hr}$$

2. Determine flow rate in gtt/min.

$$\frac{\text{(mL/hr) (gtt Factor)}}{60 \text{ minutes}} = \frac{(75)(60)}{60} = 75 \text{ gtt/min}$$

C. Calculate the flow rate in gtt/min for an IV of 500 cc to be infused over 12 hours with a set calibrated at 10 gtt/mL.

1. Determine mL/hr (or cc/hr).

$$\frac{\text{Total volume (mL or cc)}}{\text{Total time (hr)}} = \frac{500}{12} \sim 42 \text{ cc/hr}$$

2. Determine flow rate in gtt/min.

$$\frac{\text{(mL/hr) (gtt factor)}}{60 \text{ minutes}} = \frac{(42)(10)}{60} = \frac{420}{60} = 7 \text{ gtt/min}$$

D. The patient is to receive an IV medication with a volume of 20 mL in 20 minutes using a microdrip set (60 gtt/mL).

1. Determine mL/hr (20 minutes is a fractional part of an hour, $\frac{20}{60} = \frac{1}{3}$ hr).

$$\frac{\text{mL}}{\text{hr}} = \frac{20 \text{ mL}}{1/3 \text{ hr}} = 20(3/1) = 60 \text{ mL/hr}$$

2. Determine flow rate in gtt/min.

$$\frac{\text{(mL/hr) (gtt factor)}}{60 \text{ minutes}} = \frac{(60)(60)}{60} = \frac{3600}{60} = 60 \text{ gtt/min}$$

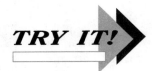

TRY IT!

PRACTICE

Calculate the flow rate for each of the IV solutions. Round answers to the nearest whole.

Order: 1000 mL to run over 12 hr
Set calibration (drop factor): 10 gtt/mL

1. _____ mL/hr

2. Flow rate: _____ gtt/min

Order: 1000 mL to run over 12 hr
Set calibration (drop factor): 60 gtt/mL (microdrip)

3. _____ mL/hr

4. Flow rate: _____ gtt/min

Order: 15 mL of IV medication to run in 30 minutes
Set calibration (drop factor): 60 gtt/mL (microdrip)

5. _____ mL/hr

6. Flow rate: _____ gtt/min

Order: 150 mL administered over 30 minutes
Set calibration (drop factor): 10 gtt/mL

7. _____ mL/hr

8. Flow rate: _____ gtt/min

Order: 500 cc to run over 6 hr
Set calibration (drop factor): 10 gtt/mL

9. _____ mL/hr

10. Flow rate: _____ gtt/min

Order: 500 mL to run over 4 hr
Set calibration (drop factor): 60 gtt/mL (microdrip)

11. _____ mL/hr

12. Flow rate: _____ gtt/min

ON THE JOB

• • • • • • • • • •

Round the answers to the nearest whole drop (gtt).

1. The physician orders 500 cc of normal saline over 8 hours. The set is calibrated at 15 gtt/mL. Calculate the flow rate in gtt/min. _____

2. Next, 500 mL of D5W (dextrose 5% in water) is ordered to infuse over 5 hours. The administration set is calibrated at 10 gtt/mL. Calculate the flow rate in gtt/min. _____

3. Then 50 cc is to be administered over 30 minutes using a microdrip set (60 gtt/mL). Calculate the flow rate in gtt/min. _____

4. If 100 cc of 10% dextrose is to be administered over 1 hour using a microdrip set (60 gtt/mL), what is the flow rate in gtt/min? _____

5. Calculate the flow rate in gtt/min when 10 mL is to be run over 30 minutes using a microdrip set (60 gtt/min). _____

Shade the given utensils to reflect the dosages indicated.

1. 18 Units U-100 insulin

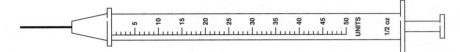

2. 0.87 cc

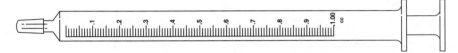

3. ℥ viii

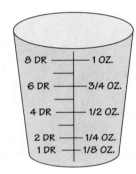

4. 1.7 mL

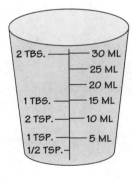

5. ℥ i

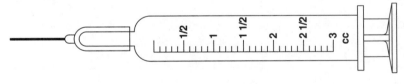

6. 57 Units U-100 insulin

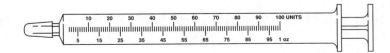

7. 1.85 cc

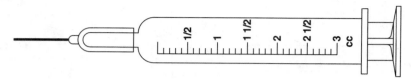

8. 0.23 cc

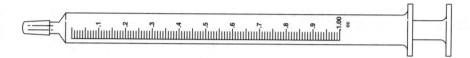

9. 6 mL

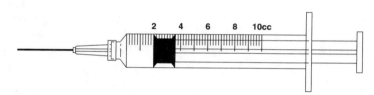

10. ℥ iv

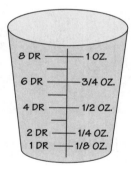

11. The supply dosage of allopurinol is 100 mg scored tablets. The physician orders gr iiss. How many tablets should be given? _____

12. Procaine penicillin, 200,000 Units, is ordered. The supply dosage is 300,000 U/mL. How many cc (to the nearest hundredth) deliver 200,000 U? _____

13. The recommended child's dosage is 30-40 mg/m². The child has a BSA of 0.62 m². What is the normal dosage range for this child? _____

14. A patient is to be given 100,000 Units. The drug label states 2.5 mL = 250,000 Units. How many cc contain 100,000 Units? _____

15. The physician ordered 250 mg of a laxative per day. The on-hand dosage is 50 mg capsules. How many capsules are to be administered in a day? _____

16. The physician orders nafcillin, 0.5 g. The dosage supply is 250 mg capsules. How many capsules should be administered? _____

17. The usual adult dose is 100 Units. What is the pediatric dose (rounded to the nearest whole unit) for a child with a BSA of 0.35 m²? _____

18. At bedtime, 30 mg of a sedative was ordered to be administered. The supply dosage is 15 mg capsules. How many capsules are to be given? _____

Interpret the following abbreviations.

19. q8h _____   20. PO _____   21. IV _____

22. q6h _____   23. NPO _____   24. OD _____

25. hs _____   26. IM _____   27. c _____

28. q _____   29. elix _____   30. R _____

31. prn _____   32. SC _____   33. ung _____

34. The physician orders penicillin, 600,000 U. The supply dosage is 500,000 U/mL. How many cc are necessary to deliver the drug order? _____

35. A physician orders meperidine HCl 37.5 mg. The vial is labeled 25 mg/1 mL. How many cc are to be injected? _____

36. A drug vial is labeled 0.25 mg = 1 cc. How many cc are necessary to deliver the drug order of 0.15 mg? _____

37. The drug order is for 0.125 mg of digoxin. The supply dosage (on-hand) is an elixir labeled 50 mcg/cc. How many cc should be administered? _____

The supply dosage of diazepam is 5 mg/mL. Calculate the volume necessary to provide the dosage ordered.

38. DRUG ORDER: 10 mg   _____

39. DRUG ORDER: 5 mg   _____

40. DRUG ORDER: 7.5 mg   _____

41. DRUG ORDER: 2 mg   _____

42. DRUG ORDER: 8 mg   _____

43. The on-hand dosage of Drug M is 0.125 mg tablets. How many tablets are to be administered if the drug order is for 250 mcg? _____

44. How many cc contain 0.08 g if the supply dosage is 10 mg/mL? _____

45. The dosage supply is digoxin elixir labeled 50 μg/cc. The drug order reads 50 mcg. How many cc should be given? _____

CHILD'S WEIGHT: 55 pounds
USUAL CHILD'S DOSAGE: 50-75 mg/kg/day in equally divided doses q 6h
SUPPLY DOSAGE: 750 mg/3 mL

46. What is the weight of the child in kilograms (to the nearest tenth, if necessary)? _____
47. What is the total daily dosage range in milligrams? _____-_____
48. What is the single dose range in milligrams to the nearest tenth? _____-_____
49. What volume (cc) is necessary to deliver a dose of 400 mg? _____

Write the appropriate abbreviation.

50. twice a day _____   51. capsule _____

52. topical _____   53. syrup _____

54. every 12 hours _____   55. with _____

56. four times a day _____   57. sublingual _____

58. solution _____   59. of each _____

60. repeat _____   61. if necessary _____

62. intravenous piggyback _____   63. freely, as desired _____

64. every _____   65. immediately _____

66. The physician ordered Drug A, 0.1 mg. The vial is labeled 0.5 mg = 2 mL. How many cc are to be administered? _____

67. A physician's order for an antibiotic is 250 mg. The capsules on-hand are 0.25 g each. How many capsules should be given to the patient? _____

68. If the drug label states that 1 mL = 40 mg, how many cc contain 0.08 g? _____

The supply dosage of heparin sodium is 1000 Units/mL. Calculate the volume necessary to provide the dosage ordered.
69. DRUG ORDER: 1800 Units _____

70. The supply dosage of phenobarbital is gr ss tablets. The physician orders gr iss. How many tablets should be given? _____

Interpret these drug orders.

71.	Roxanol	15 mg	PO	q4h	prn	
72.	meperidine HCl	50 mg tab	PO	q3-4h	prn	pain
73.	Librium	10 mg cap	PO	tid	prn	agitation
74.	Decadron	4 mg	IV	bid		
75.	morphine sulfate	8 mg	IM	q4h	prn	pain

76. If the drug label states that 2 mL contain 400 mg, how many milliliters contain 0.5 g? _____

USUAL ADULT DOSE: 300-500 mg
SUPPLY DOSAGE: 300 mg/mL
CHILD'S BSA: 0.44 m²

77. What is the dosage range for this child? (Round to the nearest tenth milligram.) _____–_____
78. What volume (cc) is necessary to deliver a 100 mg dosage? (Round to the nearest hundredth.) _____

79. What volume (cc) contains 125 mg of medication? (Round to the nearest hundredth.) _____

80. 0.25 g of a particular drug was ordered for a patient. The supply dosage is 500 mg scored tablets. How many tablets should be administered to the patient? _____

Calculate the flow rate for each of the IV solutions. Round answers to the nearest whole.
Order: 100 cc to be delivered over 1 hour
Set calibration (drop factor): 60 gtt/mL (microdrip)
81. _____ mL/hr
82. Flow rate: _____ gtt/min

Order: 110 mL to run over 1 hour
Set calibration (drop factor): 20 gtt/mL
83. _____ mL/hr
84. Flow rate: _____ gtt/min

Order: 100 mL to be delivered in 50 minutes
Set calibration (drop factor): 15 gtt/mL
85. _____ mL/hr
86. Flow rate: _____ gtt/min

Order: 150 mL to run over 3 hours
Set calibration (drop factor): 60 gtt/mL

87. _____ mL/hr
88. Flow rate: _____ gtt/min

Order: 30 mL to run over 30 minutes
Set calibration (drop factor): 15 gtt/mL

89. _____ mL/hr
90. Flow rate: _____ gtt/min

91. Initially, 1000 mL of normal saline over 16 hours is ordered. The set calibration is 10 gtt/mL. Calculate the flow rate in gtt/min. _____

92. Then 1200 mL (cc) is to be infused over a period of 10 hours. The calibration of the administration set is 20 gtt/mL. Calculate the flow rate in gtt/min. _____

93. Using a microdrip set (60 gtt/mL), 15 mL is to be administered in 20 minutes. Calculate the flow rate in gtt/min. _____

94. Normal saline, 100 cc, is to be infused over 30 minutes. The set is calibrated at 10 gtt/mL. Calculate the flow rate in gtt/min. _____

95. The physician orders 1500 mL of D5NS (dextrose 5% in normal saline) to run over 12 hours. The set calibration is 20 gtt/mL. Calculate the flow rate in gtt/min. _____